# Bisexualities and AIDS

**Social Aspects of AIDS**
*Series Editor:* Peter Aggleton
Institute of Education, University of London

*Editorial Advisory Board*

# Bisexualities and AIDS: International Perspectives

Edited by

**Peter Aggleton**

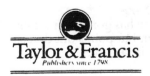

Taylor & Francis
*Publishers since 1798*

First published 1996
by Taylor & Francis
2 Park Square, Milton Park, Abingdon, Oxon, OX14 4RN

Taylor & Francis is an imprint of the Taylor & Francis Group

Transferred to Digital Printing 2006

**A Catalogue Record for this book is available from the British Library**

ISBN 0 7484 0393 0
ISBN 0 7484 0394 9 pbk

**Library of Congress Cataloging-in-Publication Data are available on request**

Series cover design by Barking Dog Art

Typeset in 10/12 pt New Baskerville
by Best-set Typesetter Ltd., Hong Kong

**Publisher's Note**
The publisher has gone to great lengths to ensure the quality of this reprint but points out that some imperfections in the original may be apparent

# Contents

Contents

# Acknowledgments

Editing this book would not have been possible without the support of numerous friends and colleagues. Within the World Health Organization's Global Programme on AIDS, where the idea for this book originated, I would like to thank Julie Dew, Purnima Mane, Eva Rodrigues, Sylvie Schaller and Oussama Tawil. Within the Institute of Education, University of London, I would like to thank Helen Thomas who liaised with chapter contributors and prepared the manuscript for publication.

Peter Aggleton

# Introduction

*Peter Aggleton*

The advent of AIDS has stimulated unprecedented interest in the nature of human sexuality and sexual behaviour, the forms that it takes and the ways in which it is understood by individuals, communities and societies. Since the first cases of AIDS were diagnosed there has been much debate about the part that male 'bisexuality' might play in fuelling the epidemic, most usually on the pretext that such behaviour in itself poses special risks, not only for the individual concerned but also for sexual partners, both male and female. But to what extent do such views offer a sound understanding of the epidemic and its determinants? And to what extent is male 'bisexuality' the same all over the world? These are important questions, not least for the design of health promotion interventions to encourage HIV-related risk reduction among behaviourally bisexual men and their partners.

In the popular media and in some medical writing, male bisexuals have often been characterized as a 'bridging group', enabling HIV to be transmitted from apparently discrete sub-populations of behaviourally homosexual and behaviourally heterosexual individuals. Most usually, it is suggested that bisexual men pose a special threat to their female partners through having had sex with other men, particularly exclusively homosexual men. Such accounts stereotype reality in that they posit the existence of two identifiable and discrete groups of individuals, the 'homosexual' and the 'heterosexual', that are capable of being 'bridged' by a third type. They also make assumptions about the nature and patterning of risk itself by implying, questionably in many circumstances, that behaviourally homosexual men are more likely to practice unsafe sex than are women and men in heterosexual sexual relations.

Male bisexuality is in fact a very complex phenomenon, especially when considered in an international and cross-cultural context. As has been emphasized elsewhere (Tielman *et al.*, 1991), important distinctions must always be drawn between bisexual behaviours and bisexual identities. While the former may be relatively common, only rarely are they accompanied by any sense of bisexual identity, or of being 'bisexual'. In fact a wide range of sexual identities accompany bisexual behaviour. Most usually, the men concerned see themselves as 'normal' and no different from other men. Alternatively and perhaps more occasionally, they may see themselves as 'partially homosexual' or as sharing one of the locally offered, and often strongly gendered, identities that allow men occasionally or even regularly to have sex with one another while retaining a strong sense of heterosexual self.

Not infrequently male bisexuality has been linked to situational factors, both as a way of explaining when and where sex takes place, and in terms of the accounts men may give of their actions. Such situational analyses can be a useful starting point in enabling us to understand sexual relations between men in environments such as prisons and the military. By themselves, however, situational analyses tend to describe rather than explain events and behaviours. As we will see here, only when complemented by in-depth study of the subjectivities of those involved and the power relations expressed by, and reproduced through, homosexual relations, do situational analyses have the strength to explain what may actually be taking place.

Few male bisexual relations are symmetrical in the sense that men apportion equally their sexual activities with women and with men, and only on the rarest of occasions is behaviour itself bisexual. Much more common are heterosexual and homosexual sexual encounters that, taken in sequence, constitute a pattern indicative of behavioural bisexuality. Such encounters are usually characterized both by an asymmetry of practice, with sexual relations with *either* women *or* men predominating at any one moment in time, and by temporal variation. Rather less is known, however, about variations in sexual identity and erotic desire that may accompany these behavioural patterns.

Any adequate understanding of male bisexuality must go beyond such relatively superficial concerns to locate bisexuality within particular cultural and historical contexts. Only this way can we fully appreciate the complex patterns it takes, as well as recurrent themes regionally and nationally. Many of the chapters here adopt such an approach, seeking to identify the roots of male bisexuality in cultural and historical variables as diverse as economic need, the social segregation of women and men, religious edict and cultural expectations about masculinity and virility. Such a mode of analysis cautions strongly against essentialist models of bisexuality and raises important questions about the attainability of any unitary bisexual politics. It points instead to the contingent and varying nature of male bisexual practice, and to its multiple determinants. Understanding more about these determinants and their consequences for HIV-related risk is central to each of the chapters in this book.

### Reference

TIELMAN, R., CARBALLO, M. and HENDRIKS, A. (Eds) (1991) *Bisexuality and HIV/AIDS*, Buffalo, NY, Prometheus.

Chapter 1

# Bisexual Men in Britain

*Mary Boulton and Ray Fitzpatrick*

Prior to the appearance of the HIV epidemic, bisexuality had received little attention from researchers in the United Kingdom. Whilst in the United States important contributions had been made to the understanding of bisexuality long before the advent of AIDS (Blumstein and Schwartz, 1976, 1977; MacDonald, 1981), in the United Kingdom bisexuality was recognized as a potential option for sexual behaviour and identity (Weeks, 1987), but little had been done to examine empirically the lives of such individuals.

An early effort to counter this lack of recognition came from individuals with bisexual biographies who collaborated in the production of collective accounts of their experiences. A number of national meetings have been held of individuals with personal interests in bisexuality, from which a very helpful volume entitled *Bisexual Lives* emerged. The book is partly a collection of personal reflections on their lives by bisexual individuals and partly a 'manifesto' of the issues facing them and the need for collective action to promote bisexual concerns and interests (Off Pink Publishing, 1988). In addition to confirming the lack of any substantial documentary evidence for bisexuality in the United Kingdom, the volume makes several fundamental points – undoubtedly observations that will appear throughout this current volume as well. Firstly, bisexual individuals are unable to find an acceptable identity for themselves from socially available straight or gay examples. Secondly, and related to the first point, they commonly experience distrust or rejection from both straight and gay communities. A third point made in a variety of ways throughout the book, however, is a quite fundamental feature of bisexuality conveyed by individuals' accounts. An extraordinary range of patterns of sexual behaviour are viewed and interpreted as bisexual. As has often been observed (Blumstein and Schwartz, 1977; Herdt, 1984), such diversity is so great as to render any essentialist approach to bisexuality profoundly problematic. Fluidity is a core feature of both personal accounts and academic commentary on bisexuality (Herdt, 1984; Rust, 1992). As the collective of authors express themselves:

> It is quite usual for the balance of a person's sexual preferences to change and evolve continuously for many reasons. Relationships may

be emotional and/or physical, contemporaneous or consecutive. The emphasis should be on a fluid sexuality rather than a fixed one. (Off Pink Publishing, 1988, pp. 5–6)

The AIDS epidemic has made it necessary to conduct applied research to monitor and model patterns of sexual behaviour and to produce explanations of behaviour to inform predictions, planning, counselling and prevention. Nevertheless bisexuality as a distinct range of experiences has been difficult to discern in much of the research in Britain as elsewhere. As this chapter makes clear, not only are individuals leading bisexual lives difficult to access for research purposes, but much of the available British evidence on HIV and bisexuality collapses categories of sexual orientation so that bisexual patterns that are distinct from gay experience are hard to discern. This chapter draws together what is known from evidence in Britain which does permit an explicit focus on bisexuality. It is concerned exclusively with bisexual men. The chapter acknowledges the fluidity of bisexuality amongst men in Britain but argues that important insights can be gained by imposing 'typological order' on such diversity and delineating distinct biographical and contextual forms of bisexuality with quite distinct implications for HIV prevention.

## The Epidemiology of Bisexuality

A primary concern of most British research in this area has been to estimate the size of the behaviourally bisexual male population and to assess the prevalence of both HIV infection and the sexual activities implicated in its transmission. Information came first from studies undertaken within the gay community, designed primarily to describe sexual behaviour and changes in sexual behaviour between men. However, these studies also showed that the majority of the men in their samples had also had sex with women at some time in their lives and that a not insignificant proportion had had a recent female partner. Thus, a number of studies reported remarkably similar findings which suggested that about 60 per cent of homosexually active men had also had lifetime sexual experience with women, and that about 10 per cent had had a female partner in the last year, and 5 per cent in the last month (McManus and McEvoy, 1987; Fitzpatrick *et al.*, 1989; Weatherburn *et al.*, 1990).

Several of these studies also provided details of the sexual activities of the men in their samples (Fitzpatrick *et al.*, 1989; Weatherburn *et al.*, 1990). Again, a remarkably consistent picture emerged, particularly concerning two key points. On the one hand, amongst those who had both male and female partners, the number of female *partners* was substantially less than the number of male partners for any given time period. On the other hand, the rates of high risk sexual *activities* with female partners were much higher than they were with male partners. Almost all men engaged in penetrative vaginal intercourse with their female partners, while only a much smaller proportion engaged in penetrative anal intercourse with male partners. Anal intercourse with female partners was not common and rates were similar to those for exclusively heterosexual men. Men were also less likely always to use condoms in penetrative sex with female compared to male partners, and more likely never to use condoms in penetrative sex with female partners. These data suggested that while men were less often engaging in high risk sex with male partners, they were continuing to engage in unsafe sex with female partners, particularly non-regular partners.

Studies of men attending genito-urinary medicine clinics presented a similar picture of the proportion of homosexually active men who also had sexual contact with women (Evans *et al.*, 1989), though uncertainty over the definition of bisexuality used and the criteria by which men were classified as homosexual or bisexual makes comparisons across studies difficult (Boulton and Coxon, 1991). Clinic studies were especially valuable, however, in providing information on the prevalence of HIV infection amongst homosexually active men classified as bisexual, particularly as government statistics used a combined category of 'homosexual/bisexual men' (e.g. PHLS Working Group, 1990). Rates of infection amongst those requesting HIV testing were reported as higher in London and the south-east than in other parts of the country. But in all testing sites and at all times, the rates of infection reported have been two to three times greater among 'homosexual' men (3 to 17 per cent) compared with 'bisexual' men (0.7 to 10 per cent) (Welch *et al.*, 1986; Joshi *et al.*, 1988; Collaborative Study Group, 1989). In one particularly detailed study of over a thousand homosexual and bisexual men attending a London clinic and wanting an HIV test, rates of infection declined as men were more 'actively bisexual': 30 per cent of homosexual men tested HIV positive, while the rate of infection amongst men who had had a female partner in the last year was only 12 per cent and amongst those who had had a female partner in the last month as low as 5 per cent (Evans *et al.*, 1989).

The consistency of the finding that rates of HIV infection were lower amongst bisexual than exclusively homosexual men led to the suggestion that gay and bisexual men might constitute distinct populations (Evans *et al.*, 1989). Distinctive social characteristics have been noted in several studies, which report that bisexual men are more likely than exclusively homosexual men to be, or have been, married and more likely to be young (Davies *et al.*, 1990) and middle-class (Fitzpatrick *et al.*, 1989). Nevertheless, these same studies found few differences in attitudes and behaviour between exclusively homosexual and bisexual men. For example, Fitzpatrick *et al.* (1989) found that bisexual men were just as likely as gay men to have been the active partner in anal sex with a man and only slightly less likely to have been the passive partner. Most notably in relation to risk of HIV infection, the histories of sexually transmitted diseases were similar in the two groups.

The last and potentially most compelling source of information on the population prevalence of behaviourally bisexual men is the National Survey of Sexual Attitudes and Lifestyles (NSSAL) (Johnson *et al.*, 1994). A fundamental limitation of both clinic-based studies and surveys within the gay community is the unknown relationship between their samples and the populations from which they are drawn. This makes generalizations from their findings problematic. The NSSAL is important in providing detailed information on the sexual behaviour of a representative sample of the population as a whole. The researchers took a stratified random sample of almost 20,000 households and obtained information from over 8,000 men (65 per cent response rate). Data were collected through both face-to-face interviews and confidential self-completed booklets. The study found that 6.1 per cent of men reported having had 'any homosexual experience' ever and 3.6 per cent a homosexual partner involving genital contact. However, only 1.4 per cent reported a homosexual partner in the last five years and 1.1 per cent in the last year. The research team also found that exclusively homosexual experience was rare. Of the men who reported ever having had a male partner, 90.3 per cent had also had a female partner; of those who had had a male partner in the last five years, 58.4 per cent had also had a female partner; and of those who had had a male partner in the last year, 29.9 per cent had also had a female partner. In comparison with studies conducted in the gay community, these figures show a substantially higher proportion of homosexually active men as also having a female sexual partner: for the last year, the rate is three times as high. This may be because the NSSAL has recruited from a slightly different population of homosexually active men. In particular, it is likely that the NSSAL has included a higher proportion of non-gay-identified men who have female sexual partners but who also engage in covert sex with men than were included in gay community studies, whose samples were drawn largely from amongst 'out' gay men. If this is the case, then the implication is that the great majority of behaviourally bisexual men are not involved in the gay community.

Overall, the proportion of men in the survey who reported both male and female partners was 3.4 per cent ever, 0.8 per cent in the last five years, and 0.4 per cent in the last year. These figures are low but consistent with those reported by national surveys conducted using very different methods in both Norway (Sundet *et al.*, 1988) and France (ACSF Investigators, 1992). As the only ones available based on a random sample of the population, these figures are likely to gain wide acceptance as the 'official' statistics for Britain. Nevertheless, they have been met by considerable surprise and scepticism, particularly by those involved in the gay community who maintain that they substantially under-represent the proportion of homosexually active men. Weatherburn and Davies (1993), for example, argue that there are a number of methodological reasons why the NSSAL is likely to give an underestimate of the homosexually active male population and hence the behaviourally bisexual population. They consider the findings of several surveys conducted in the 'heterosexually identified population' in the USA and settle for much higher estimates of homosexual activity. With regard to the prevalence of bisexual behaviour, they suggest that between 5 and 15 per cent of 'heterosexually identified men' are behaviourally bisexual at some point in their lives and between 1 and 2 per cent are behaviourally bisexual in any given year.

This debate points to some of the problems inherent in survey research on behaviourally bisexual men. On the one hand, large-scale population surveys inevitably have difficulty in recruiting appropriate numbers of individuals involved in stigmatized or covert activities and may have further problems in eliciting accurate information from them. The population estimates they give are therefore open to question. On the other hand, studies conducted in the gay community are likely to exclude non-gay-identified men and to view questions to do with bisexuality from a gay perspective. The picture they present is thus again limited and potentially misleading. Few studies have attempted to recruit behaviourally bisexual men directly, however, as the absence of significant social institutions to draw them together leaves such men as inaccessible to research as they are invisible to the public in general.

### The Complexity of Bisexuality

The public health concerns which have underpinned much of the survey research on sexuality in the last decade or so have served to focus attention largely on sexual *behaviour*. To some extent, this represents the success of social scientists in making clear the distinction between sexual behaviour and social labels and in underlining the need to look specifically at behaviour (and the details of sexual activities) to understand the epidemiology of HIV/AIDS. A focus on behaviour alone, however, can present only a partial and limited picture of sexuality. This is particularly evident in relation to bisexuality, where different dimensions of sexuality have been shown to bear no straightforward relationship to one another. Thus, it has frequently been observed that considerably more men report sexual contact with both male and female partners than describe themselves as bisexual and, in turn, that considerably more men report sexual attractions to both men and women than express this in sexual contact with male and female partners (Boulton and Weatherburn, 1990).

A clearer picture of the complexity and dimensionality of bisexuality can be seen in a longitudinal study conducted by ourselves and other colleagues to investigate the sexual behaviour and changes in behaviour of homosexually active men in relation to HIV/AIDS (Fitzpatrick *et al.*, 1989, 1990a). A cohort of 502 men who had had sex with a male partner in the previous five years were recruited from gay pubs, clubs and organizations and from genitourinary medicine clinics. As in most studies of gay and homosexual males, the men were fairly young (mean age 31.6 years, SD 10.4) and well educated (63 per cent having some form of higher or further education). The men were asked about a wide range of topics, including details of their partners in the previous year, the term they would use to describe their sexual orientation, and their sexual fantasies and attractions rated on the Kinsey scale, from exclusively heterosexual through equally heterosexual and homosexual to exclusively homosexual. The study found that 495 (99 per cent) of the men had had a male partner and 58 (12 per cent) had had a female partner in the year prior to interview. Most men (435, 87 per cent) described themselves as gay or homosexual, 51 (10 per cent) described themselves as bisexual and the remaining 16 (3 per cent) preferred none of these terms. Over a third (184, 37 per cent) described some degree of heterosexual fantasies and attractions, the rest (318, 63 per cent) exclusively homosexual fantasies and attractions.

Comparing the men's *behaviour* with their ratings of their sexual *attractions*, 30 per cent (133/444) of the men who had not had sex with a female partner in the previous year nonetheless described some degree of heterosexual attraction, while 12 per cent (7/58) of those who had had a female sexual partner described their attractions as exclusively homosexual. Discontinuities were also found when men's behaviour was compared with their self-ascribed sexual orientation: 4 per cent (17/444) of men who had not had a female partner in the previous year nonetheless described themselves as bisexual, while almost half (43 per cent, 25/58) of those who had had a female partner did *not* describe themselves as bisexual. Finally, self-ascribed sexual orientation and ratings of sexual fantasies and attraction again did not match up neatly. In particular, of the 392 who referred to themselves as gay, 105 (27 per cent) chose a point on the Kinsey scale that indicated some degree of heterosexual attraction.

These men were then followed up nine months later with a postal questionnaire. Three-quarters of the men (369, 74 per cent) responded, allowing comparisons to be made over time for at least a proportion of the sample. In relation to sexual behaviour, 46 men reported having sex with a male and female partner in the previous year in response to the questions in *either* the first *or* the second questionnaire. However, only 14 men (14/46, 30 per cent) reported sexual contact with a male and female partner in response to *both* questionnaires. Similarly, 39 men described their sexual orientation as bisexual in response to the questions in at least one of the two questionnaires. Only half (20/39, 51 per cent) of the men, however, were consistent in describing themselves as bisexual in response to *both* questionnaires.

Thus, it is clear that bisexuality is both complex and fluid. It involves at least three dimensions of behaviour, attractions and sexual orientation or identity. These dimensions do not map on to one another in any simple or straightforward way, either at one point in time or predictively over time. And no single dimension can alone adequately capture its nature or quality.

### Identity or Image: How Do Behaviourally Bisexual Men See Themselves?

To explore further the complexity of bisexuality, we conducted a second, more 'in-depth' study of the views, experience and behaviour of a sample of behaviourally bisexual men (Boulton and Coxon, 1991). Sixty men were recruited to the study using snowballing techniques from the previous study, placing advertisements in appropriate magazines, through genito-urinary medicine clinics and via bisexual groups in London and Edinburgh. The sample was again fairly young and middle-class: the mean age was 34 years with a range from 19 to 71 and two-thirds had non-manual occupations.

All the men in the study had had male and female partners at some time in the previous five years and almost all expected to have both male and female partners in the future. Using the Kinsey scale, almost all (56, 93 per cent) also described their fantasies and attractions as to some degree both homosexual and heterosexual, and two-thirds (39, 65 per cent) described them as more or less *equally* homosexual and heterosexual. When asked how they would describe themselves, however, only half (34, 57 per cent) of the men used the term bisexual. A quarter (13, 22 per cent) said gay, 4 (7 per cent) said straight and the remaining 9 (15 per cent) used a variety of other terms such as 'normal' and 'unrestrained'. Moreover, even those who used the term bisexual did so in a purely descriptive sense:

> I would normally try to avoid labelling myself as much as labelling others, I suppose I thought 'OK, obviously I've got homosexual tendencies to which I'm giving expression, and I've also got heterosexual tendencies and I'm having relations both ways, so perhaps I'm bisexual if I have to put a term on it.' I didn't go off and check what that meant in the dictionary. Expressing my sexuality was just one of many things I was wanting and doing at that time and since.

Thus, men who could reasonably be described as bisexual in terms of both their attractions and behaviour often did not think of themselves as bisexual. With only a few exceptions, even amongst those who did accept it as an accurate description of themselves, the men did not use the term bisexual to refer to essential aspects of their selves. It did not provide them with an 'identity' in terms of which they organized and interpreted key aspects of their lives as, for example, a gay identity did for others in the study. This, we would suggest, is at least in part because no significant social organization or cohesive political structures have yet emerged to provide a focal point for the development of a distinctive bisexual community and the stabilization of a distinct bisexual identity (George *et al.*, 1993). Furthermore, in Britain, as in other Western countries, dichotomous notions of sexuality continue to predominate (Boulton and Weatherburn, 1990). Within the wider society, any same-sex sexual activity is seen as marking an individual out as 'homosexual', while within gay culture heterosexual behaviour is frowned on as self-deceptive or disloyal and bisexual behaviour is again not seen as legitimate. The politics of gay liberation have to some extent opened up the possibilities of bisexual behaviour but sanctions within both the heterosexual and gay communities act to push individuals to commit themselves to one community or the other.

It is perhaps not surprising, then, that very few men (11, 18 per cent) thought that *other* people saw them as bisexual. This is in part because the stigma attached to homosexual sex meant that a number of men were concerned to keep it hidden from view or content to allow it to remain publicly invisible:

> How do other people see me? They see me as a straight man because I make very sure they do.

> The majority of people see me as a straight man. That's the assumption they make because I'm married and have children.

However, even those who were open about their sexual preferences felt that sexual contact with both men and women did not necessarily mean that they were defined as bisexual by others. Most men said that others saw them as either heterosexual (32, 53 per cent) or as gay (8, 13 per cent), whatever their sexual attractions and partners:

> People close to me, my close friends, know that I sleep with men. They know I've got a long-term partner. . . . No, they wouldn't see me as bisexual, but as someone who's straight but who also sleeps with men as well.

> I work in a gay café, I socialize mostly with gay people. People know I have had, and would in the future have, relationships with women. I still class myself, refer to myself as a gay man. It's a political classification. I am a gay man and I am known as a gay man.

The men's views of themselves were thus reflected in and reinforced by the views of those around them. These views might recognize 'bisexual' as an accurate description of behaviour, but they did not allow it as a legitimate personal identity nor a viable social category. For some, this meant living with a fragmented and conflicting view of themselves:

> My family think of me as heterosexual because that's one of the things in life, you don't always come out to your family. A number of my friends who only know me on the gay side think of me as gay, yet other friends think of me as bisexual. . . . The balance must come in favour of bisexual, though because I have a gay lover that I have lived

with for years, they would say bisexual but living a gay life. That's how they think of me.

Some people think I'm gay, others think bisexual. It doesn't bother me that people think differently about me.

Those people who do not know my sexual inclinations assume that I'm heterosexual. Those homosexual friends that I have, because I'm married, assume that I'm bisexual. They wouldn't allow that I am not homosexual but I'm married so I must be bisexual.

Few men, however, found this problematic or tried to pull the strands of their lives together around a more coherent ideology. With the exception of those recruited via bisexual groups, bisexuality rarely provided a point of reference for the men and few sought out other bisexual individuals to support a bisexual identity or lifestyle. Instead, most men took a fairly individualistic view of their sexual identity and a fairly pragmatic approach to their social lives. They moved between the gay and straight communities, drawing on each as it suited them, and seemed to prefer doing so to joining a third, bisexual community. They felt little collective solidarity with other bisexuals and little concern for the public acceptance of bisexuality so long as they themselves could continue to have both male and female partners.

### The Temporal Diversity of Bisexuality

Thus, for many men involved in sexual activities with men and women, bisexuality is a term that captures and summarizes personal *biography* rather than an expression of personal *identity* or *identification* with a social or political group. The most significant features of personal biography so captured are, of course, sexual relationships or emotional attachments to both men and women. However, it is striking how diverse are the temporal spans and range of possible sequences of male and female sexual relations that are encompassed by individuals to whom the term may reasonably be applied. Six very distinct patterns of sexual history were found in our in-depth study of bisexuality. The first three patterns in particular do not involve any of the concurrent homosexual and bisexual sexual activities that are most commonly associated in popular imagination with bisexuality and the term only applies if a more diachronic approach to sexual history is adopted.

The first pattern was termed 'transitional' and reflects the process of 'coming out' as gay. Men to whom this term applied were in transition from exclusively or predominantly heterosexual activity and, at the time of interview, regarded themselves as gay and intending to be exclusively homosexual in their current sexual activities. Thus a 30-year-old librarian had lived with a girlfriend for several years whilst at university. He had had several subsequent girlfriends, one of whom he described as bisexual. She had encouraged him to explore his own homosexual feelings. At the time of interview he lived with a male lover and had had other regular and casual male partners in the previous five years.

A second pattern was defined as 'unique'. This term was applied to men who were otherwise involved in exclusively homosexual or heterosexual sexual activity but who 'deviated' from this pattern on just one or two occasions. Several men described a situation involving drugs or alcohol as inducing this aberrant episode. For a few men the deviant sexual relationship was a physical expression of emotional involvement in one special friend. A 23-year-old labourer who had a steady girlfriend also became involved in a sexual relationship with his best male friend for several years. After this friend was killed in a motor accident, he had not felt attracted to any other men. All of the men to whose biographies the term 'unique' applies viewed their identities as gay or straight as unaffected by the 'deviant' relationship.

A third and less common pattern was termed 'serial' to reflect a pattern in which men were involved in non-overlapping homosexual and heterosexual relationships. A 26-year-old telephone technician currently lived with a regular male partner. However, he described non-overlapping, monogamous relationships with four male and three female partners in the six-year period prior to the interview. Generally speaking, the small number of men who conformed to this pattern had fewer partners overall than men in other groups.

The majority of bisexual men in our study show a pattern of overlapping homosexual and heterosexual activities that is easier to associate with popular imagery of bisexuality. Nevertheless different forms of concurrent bisexuality can be distinguished by reference to the very diverse social contexts in which men lived.

The fourth pattern of bisexuality is termed 'concurrent straight'. Men are here involved in relationships with women (usually a wife or long-term female partner) but have male partners at the same time. A 43-year-old businessman is typical of men in this group. He lived with his wife but had had over sixty male partners in the year prior to being interviewed for our study. His wife was aware of his past homosexual activity, but not of his current male partners since he had agreed to stop having homosexual sex after their marriage. Amongst the men in this group, numbers of male partners were considerably higher than numbers of female partners and many men had just one female partner.

A fifth pattern, 'concurrent gay', is in many ways the mirror image of the fourth pattern. Men here lead open and active lives in gay culture but regularly also have sexual relationships with women. Amongst men in this group, approximately equal numbers of men described themselves as gay or bisexual. An important difference between this and the 'concurrent straight' bisexual pattern is that the women involved generally were aware of their partner's homosexual activity.

A sixth and relatively uncommon pattern was 'concurrent opportunistic'. These men were not in long-term stable relationships, but had sex opportunistically with either men or women. As an illustration, a 20-year-old hotelier described several regular and casual female partners that he had met in the last year through his work or at parties. At the same time he regularly used contact magazines to meet other men for casual sex.

The typology of patterns of bisexuality does not include some of the forms that Gagnon (1989) distinguishes. In particular he notes from American ethnographic work forms of bisexuality that may be termed situational: men who would otherwise be heterosexually active but who are constrained by circumstances towards homosexual sexual activity. Two situations in particular are identified: homosexual sex arising from the constraints of incarceration and homosexual sex arising from male prostitution for economic reasons. These two patterns are inherently difficult to research for legal reasons. There is some research evidence of homosexual prostitution but it provides little detail of the extent of heterosexual sex outside client transactions that male escorts, masseurs and streetwalkers have (Davies and Simpson, 1990).

### Varying Contexts for Bisexuality

It will be clear from the previous section that men may lead bisexual lives in quite different social contexts. It is possible analytically to distinguish three such social contexts from our in-depth study: heterosexual, bisexual and gay. Men were considered to be embedded in a heterosexual context if they were married or living with a female or identified themselves as heterosexual. Men were considered to be embedded in a gay context if they were significantly involved in the organized gay community, for example belonging to gay organizations and regularly using gay pubs and clubs. The third, bisexual context applies to those men who describe themselves as bisexual and had been recruited via the organized bisexual community. The sample is too small to attach too much significance to numerical data. However, nearly half of the sample (29, 48 per cent) were embedded in a heterosexual context, whilst a quarter (15, 25 per cent) were in a gay context and another quarter (13, 22 per cent) in a bisexual context. Three men in the sample were too marginal to any social context to be classified in this way.

Several important differences were noted in the sexual behaviour of men in the three different contexts, although, again, numbers are too small for confidence to be placed in the significance of differences. In the first place, men in bisexual contexts were *less* likely to have had unprotected penetrative sex with male or female partners in the last year; 77 per cent (10/13) in a bisexual context reported no unprotected penetrative sex compared with 31 per cent (9/29) in heterosexual contexts and 40 per cent (6/15) in gay contexts. It appeared to be the norm to practise safer sex in the group identified as in a bisexual context. It is only possible to speculate that greater openness to women about their homosexual activities is facilitated by an explicitly bisexual context and that safer sex is a consequence or concomitant of such openness.

A second difference was also noted. Men in a heterosexual context were less likely than men in a gay context (28 per cent, 8/29, as against 53 per cent, 8/15) to have unprotected penetrative sex with their male partners. One possible reason for these differences is that men living in a heterosexual context – that is, in a regular relationship with a female partner – were less likely to have a regular male partner. There is considerable evidence that a relationship with a regular partner is one of the most important of circumstances facilitating unprotected penetrative sex amongst gay men (Fitzpatrick *et al.*, 1990a, 1990b; McLean *et al.*, 1994). It may also be the case that men in this study living in a heterosexual context felt that safer sex was more likely to allow them to maintain their sexual activity with men as a secret from their female partners, for example by keeping them free from sexually transmitted diseases of any sort.

A final difference to be noted is that men in heterosexual contexts were more likely to have unprotected penetrative sex with female partners (55 per cent, 16/29) compared with men in gay contexts (20 per cent, 3/15). One possible explanation for these differences is that the use of a condom in the context of a 'straight' heterosexual relationship would require an explanation for unusual behaviour and, in some cases, jeopardize the secrecy of other concurrent homosexual relationships. The need to control information and cues regarding sexual history arose for a number of reasons that the next section explores further.

### Bisexuality and Information Control

For a majority of men in the in-depth study, bisexuality was something requiring considerable efforts to control the flow of information about their sexual biography. This arose for two quite distinct reasons. On the one hand they viewed bisexuality as a problematic state. It involved 'felt stigma' (Scambler and Hopkins, 1986); in other words, a sense of being different from and unacceptable to wider society even though they experienced few if any occasions of 'enacted stigma', direct discrimination from the wider society. On the other hand, concealing or managing information about past or current sexual behaviour was a frequent necessity in maintaining relationships particularly in terms of controlling evidence of homosexual activities from female partners.

As has been noted for many other kinds of problematic social labels (Goffman, 1968; Scambler, 1984), the grounds for feeling stigmatized were difficult for men to express precisely but none the less strongly felt. The commonest observation made by men was how ignorant society was of the very existence of bisexuality. As one man observed:

> I think they think you're either gay or you're not. There's a lot of naivety, so I would say they're not aware of bisexuality.

This view was commonly echoed in other men's reflections of society's difficulties in viewing alternatives to gay or straight identity:

> They accept homosexuality more because it's an identity. And they don't class bisexuality as an identity. A lot of straight guys would say: 'You're either gay or you're straight. You can't be both.'

This observation gives some indication of how lack of public awareness shades into lack of acceptance. Society is seen as having a dichotomous conception of sexual identity. It not only cannot accept but is also threatened by bisexuality. As one man observed:

> Bisexuality involves acceptance of 'otherness' existing in the normal married man. It's much more threatening to the neatness of family life. Gay men just don't exist in this sense for the general public.

Or in another rather graphic explanation:

> I think straight men see gay men as definitely different, as over the fence, separate from us, the healthy men. They are like animals in a zoo and we go and look at them sometimes. Bisexual men are closer to straight men and share the straight world and are therefore more difficult to cope with. They can't be distanced so easily.

Lack of acceptance, in their view, was also related to public envy of bisexuals for 'having it both ways', and also, in a phrase frequently used in the sample, to their role as a 'bridging group' for HIV (Boulton and Fitzpatrick, 1993).

For a variety of reasons, therefore, men involved in bisexual activity expected negative responses from others to their sexual biography and took steps to conceal their bisexuality when necessary. However, the problem also arose in the course of managing and maintaining relationships. Men did not feel that their male partners were particularly concerned to discover their history of female sexual partners. The situation was very different with female partners. They expected women to be shocked or indeed disgusted by the idea of male homosexual sex. As one man said of women's attitudes in general:

> They think it's disgusting, men together and especially anal sex. They think it's dirty.

Alternatively men feared that women would view male partners who were also involved in gay sex as unreliable or untrustworthy:

The general view is that bisexuals get married but then go out and continue to have sex with men, so they make unsatisfactory husbands and fathers. Basically they are not to be trusted.

For these reasons men often went to great lengths to conceal their bisexual history from female partners. Some maintained that their wives had no idea about their homosexual activities. Such concealment generally required very elaborate efforts to keep separate their concurrent contact with male partners and an otherwise heterosexual lifestyle. If their homosexual activities were historical, concealment usually was achieved because the subject need not arise with new regular female partners:

We never got into the situation, sitting around in bars or hotels, of having deep discussions about people being gay or whatever. I didn't keep anything from her by lying, but she would have assumed I was straight.

Some men preferred to reveal *past* homosexual activities but to conceal any continuing homosexual activities:

She certainly knew about my male partners before I started going out with her. She didn't know that I was having sex with men while I was seeing her. I kept that quiet. What a toad I am!

At the other extreme men would reveal their bisexual activities to women completely. This approach tended to be commonest amongst men living in a bisexual context and committed to an open bisexual lifestyle. In a small number of cases this was facilitated by the fact that a female partner was also bisexual. However, more commonly female partners did not share their bisexual lifestyle and revelation of the individual's bisexual history had negative consequences for the relationship:

I told her that I was attracted to men before I ever slept with a man. She said she wasn't surprised. It took a lot of courage because I knew I was spelling end of the relationship. It was a very close relationship and she didn't want it to involve anyone else.

Again the exact nature of the risks men felt to their relationships with women are unclear. It is likely that female partners would become more concerned about risks of HIV if they discovered their partner also had homosexual sex; however men also feared a more general negative reaction:

If I was having penetrative sex with men, she wouldn't do it with me. We didn't discuss whether that was to do with AIDS. It might have been that she found it disgusting.

All of the above concerns about whether to reveal bisexual activities were far less likely to arise when female partners were part of either casual or short-lived relationships. This may be because of simple pragmatism and the lack of any felt need for establishing trust and mutuality from openness in such encounters.

### Risk Perception and Partner Perception

Studies of sexual behaviour in the context of AIDS have taken some time to free themselves from the limitations of psychological models largely developed to understand behaviour arising from non-infectious chronic diseases (Dawson *et al.*, 1992). Approaches such as the Health Belief Model emphasized the influence on health behaviour of actors' perceptions of their own level of susceptibility to a particular health problem such as heart disease, cancer or other chronic diseases. In the context of a virus that may be transmitted sexually from other individuals, it will be perceptions of *other* individuals' 'riskiness' that are more important. It is also clear that such perceptions are not particularly strongly determined by knowledge of sexual partners' HIV status (McLean *et al.*, 1994). A variety of indirect and indeed irrelevant cues are relied upon as evidence that someone is unlikely to be HIV positive (Gold and Skinner, 1992; Levine and Siegel, 1992). The other weakness of many available models of health behaviour has been that sexual behaviour primarily involves interpersonal attraction and emotions such as love, desire and trust, factors unconcerned with perceptions of health risk. It has proved essential to develop explanations of sexual behaviour in relation to HIV that more directly address such factors.

Bisexual men's sexual behaviour also needs to be understood in the context of perceptions of risk from partners on the one hand and emotional factors such as desire and attachment on the other hand. It was clear that men generally did not consider themselves at risk of HIV infection from female partners. This was mainly said to be because very few women were HIV positive. Many men also added that, whatever the general levels of HIV infection in women, their own partners were perceived to be at low risk. This involved a certain level of stereotypic thinking. For example a 32-year-old computer programmer explained his views thus:

> Even in Edinburgh, the kind of women I would sleep with, I wouldn't expect to sleep with any drug-addicted women. I suppose there's the assumption on my part that I'm sleeping with low-risk women compared to some of the women in Edinburgh.

By contrast the female partners of bisexual men had more diverse views, as reported by their partners. Some women clearly were concerned about their bisexual male partners, in some cases insisting on monogamy and a negative HIV test as a condition for continuing relationships. A 27-year-old engineer explained his arrangements thus:

> We've discussed this and that's why I don't have sex with men any more, because we do see it as a problem. My wife was very worried about me and about herself. She wanted me to have an HIV test, which I did.

Other female partners were described as having no concerns in this regard. One man described the views of his female partners generally in these terms:

> Women are generally warier now than they were before because they know about risk groups, but they don't demand condoms. They are less concerned than men are and they're prepared to let me take responsibility.

The most obvious factor that appears to influence such perceptions is whether or not the female partner is aware of her male partner's homosexual activities.

Men's perceptions of being at low risk from women contrasted markedly with their perceptions and behaviour with male partners. As has already been explained, men recognized the potential for risk, especially with casual partners, and took appropriate precautions.

### Implications for HIV Prevention

On the surface, the evidence reviewed in this chapter might be viewed as posing a rather too daunting challenge in terms of AIDS/HIV prevention. What little public discussion has occurred in the United Kingdom regarding bisexuality has adopted the rather simplistic notion of a single 'bridging group', which, once identified, could be targeted for preventive interventions. It is clear that there is no such homogeneous social group who might be reached in any simple sense. There is a remarkable diversity of social contexts and personal biographies that may be meaningfully considered as bisexual. It was always just as naive to assume that there would be a 'bisexual community' that could be targeted as to hope that all homosexually active men would be reached via the 'gay community'. Not only is there substantial diversity. Many men with bisexual sexual histories do not view themselves as bisexual and do not take any part in social or political activities that concern bisexuality.

It is perhaps not surprising, then, that bisexual men have been largely overlooked within the realm of HIV prevention activities in Britain. A survey of relevant agencies, including both voluntary gay and bisexual organizations and statutory HIV/AIDS prevention coordinators, revealed that at a local level very little work was being done on bisexual issues (George *et al.*, 1993). Somewhat more progress has been made in relation to national media campaigns developed by the Health Education Authority (HEA, 1994). The needs of bisexual men are considered in the design of campaigns targeted at both 'out' gay men and the 'heterosexually identified' general population and two advertisements, which appear in general 'lifestyle' magazines, are aimed specifically at men who have both male and female sexual partners. They are of particular value in putting bisexuality firmly and explicitly on the public agenda. However, they draw on the common stereotypes of bisexual men: the married (homosexual) man who has (secret) affairs with men and the young man who is 'uncertain' of his sexuality. While the images they present are arresting and attractive, they are limited in the possibilities they acknowledge and once again reflect and reinforce an implicit notion that 'true' sexuality is *either* homosexual *or* heterosexual.

What the evidence reviewed in this chapter makes very clear is that bisexual sexual behaviour is considerably more fluid and diverse than such notions would allow. Nonetheless, the apparently overwhelming variability of bisexual sexual behaviour can be understood in terms of a finite and more manageable range of contexts that can be targeted via health education and health promotion. The cognitive, emotional and social processes involved in sexual activities amongst bisexual men are in many ways no different from those prevailing amongst other social groups. Our research has revealed themes in bisexual lives such as optimistic bias, stereotypic thinking, the dilemmas of trust in relationships, and the difficulties of balancing emotional needs with health considerations that can be all explicitly addressed via imaginative campaigns of general relevance.

There are particular problems of information control that men maintain in some bisexual contexts that may also be addressed by conceiving of interventions from the partner's perspective; in other words, increasing general awareness of the diversity of sexual histories via health promotion campaigns may make some contribution to changing potentially harmful asymmetries of information.

Overall there are grounds for optimism. There is no evidence that rates of HIV infection have deteriorated amongst bisexually active men. Patterns of bisexual sexual behaviour, in so far as it is possible accurately to monitor them, also offer grounds for optimism. The same careful balance is required as in the case of gay men: on the one hand, being impressed and encouraged by positive social and behavioural responses to the challenge of HIV, and, on the other hand, alertness and imagination in addressing risks arising from sexual behaviour.

### Note

We would like to acknowledge the contribution of our colleagues Graham Hart, Jill Dawson, John McLean and Zoe Schramm-Evans in carrying out the research on gay and bisexual men described in this chapter. We would also like to thank the Medical Research Council and the Economic and Social Research Council for funding the work.

### References

ACSF INVESTIGATORS (1992) 'AIDS and Sexual Behaviour in France', *Nature*, 360, pp. 407–9.

BLUMSTEIN, P. and SCHWARTZ, P. (1976) 'Bisexuality in Men', *Urban Life*, 5, pp. 339–58.

BLUMSTEIN, P. and SCHWARTZ, P. (1977) 'Bisexuality: Some Social Psychological Issues', *Journal of Social Issues*, 33, pp. 30–45.

BOULTON, M. (1991) 'Review of the Literature on Bisexuality and HIV Transmission', in TIELMAN, R., CARBALLO, M. and HENDRIKS, A. (Eds) *Bisexuality and HIV/AIDS: A Global Perspective*, New York, Prometheus.

BOULTON, M. and COXON, T. (1991) 'Bisexuality in the United Kingdom', in TIELMAN, R., CARBALLO, M. and HENDRIKS, A. (Eds) *Bisexuality and HIV/AIDS: A Global Perspective*, New York, Prometheus Books.

BOULTON, M. and FITZPATRICK, R. (1993) 'The Public and Personal Meanings of Bisexuality in the Context of AIDS', in ALBRECHT, G. and ZIMMERMAN, R. (Eds) *The Social and Behavioural Aspects of AIDS. Advances in Medical Sociology*, 3, Greenwich, Conn., JAI Press.

BOULTON, M. and WEATHERBURN, P. (1990) 'Literature Review on Bisexuality and HIV Transmission', report commissioned by the Global Programme on AIDS, World Health Organization.

BOULTON, M., SCHRAMM-EVANS, Z., FITZPATRICK, R. and HART, G. (1991) 'Bisexual Men: Women, Safer Sex and HIV Transmission', in AGGLETON, P., DAVIES, P. and HART, G. (Eds) *AIDS: Responses, Interventions and Care*, London, Falmer Press.

BOULTON, M., HART, G. and FITZPATRICK, R. (1992) 'The Sexual Behaviour of Bisexual Men in Relation to HIV Transmission', *AIDS Care*, 4, pp. 165–75.

COLLABORATIVE STUDY GROUP OF CONSULTANTS IN GU MEDICINE AND THE PUBLIC HEALTH LABORATORY SERVICE (1989) 'HIV Infection in Patients Attending Clinics for Sexually Transmitted Diseases in England and Wales', *British Medical Journal*, 298, pp. 415–18.

DAVIES, P. and SIMPSON, P. (1990) 'On Male Homosexual Prostitution', in AGGLETON, P., DAVIES, P. and HART, G. (Eds) *AIDS: Individual, Cultural and Policy Dimensions*, Basingstoke, Falmer Press.

DAVIES, P., HUNT, A., MACOURT, M. and WEATHERBURN, P. (1990) 'Longitudinal Study of Sexual Behaviour of Homosexually Active Males under the Impact of AIDS', Project SIGMA, Final Report to the Department of Health.

DAWSON, J., FITZPATRICK, R., BOULTON, M., McLEAN, J. and HART, G. (1992) 'Predictors of High Risk Sexual Behaviour in Gay and Bisexual Men', *Sozial und Präventivmedizin*, 37, pp. 79–84.

EVANS, B., MCLEAN, K., DAWSON, S. *et al.* (1989) 'Trends in Sexual Behaviour and Risk Factors for HIV Infection among Homosexual Men', *British Medical Journal*, 298, pp. 215–18.

FITZPATRICK, R., HART, G., BOULTON, M., MCLEAN, J. and DAWSON, J. (1989) 'Heterosexual Sexual Behaviour in a Sample of Homosexually Active Men', *Genitourinary Medicine*, 65, pp. 259–62.

FITZPATRICK, R., MCLEAN, J., DAWSON, J., BOULTON, M. and HART, G. (1990a) 'Factors Influencing Condom Use in a Sample of Homosexually Active Men', *Genitourinary Medicine*, 66, pp. 346–50.

FITZPATRICK, R., MCLEAN, J., BOULTON, M., HART, G. and DAWSON, J. (1990b) 'Variation in Sexual Behaviour in Gay Men', in AGGLETON, P., DAVIES, P. and HART, G. (Eds) *AIDS: Individual, Cultural and Policy Dimensions*, Basingstoke, Falmer Press.

GAGNON, J. (1989) 'Disease and Desire', *Daedalus*, 118, pp. 47–78.

GEORGE, S., DEYNEM, H., FARQUHARSON, P., WILLIAMS, G. and BURKLE, D. (1993) *Bisexuality and HIV Prevention*, London, Health Education Authority.

GOFFMAN, E. (1968) *Stigma*, Harmondsworth, Penguin Books.

GOLD, R. and SKINNER, M. (1992) 'Situational Factors and Thought Processes Associated with Unprotected Intercourse in Young Gay Men', *AIDS*, 6, pp. 1021–30.

HEALTH EDUCATION AUTHORITY (1994) Gay/Bisexual Press Advertising Campaign 1994/4 (internal document).

HERDT, G. (1984) 'A Comment on Cultural Attributes and Fluidity of Bisexuality', *Journal of Homosexuality*, 10, pp. 53–61.

JOHNSON, A., WADSWORTH, J., WELLINGS, K., FIELD, J. and BRADSHAW, S. (1994) *Sexual Attitudes and Lifestyles*, Oxford, Blackwell Scientific Publications.

JOSHI, U., CAMERON, S., SOMMERVILLE, J. and SOMMERVILLE, R. (1988) 'HIV Testing in Glasgow Genito-Urinary Medicine Clinics 1985–1987', *Scottish Medical Journal*, 33, pp. 294–5.

LEVINE, M. and SIEGEL, K. (1992) 'Unprotected Sex: Understanding Gay Men's Participation', in HUBER, J. and SCHEIDER, B. (Eds) *The Social Context of AIDS*, London, Sage.

MACDONALD, A. (1981) 'Bisexuality: Some Comments on Research and Theory', *Journal of Homosexuality*, 6, pp. 21–36.

MCLEAN, J., BOULTON, M., BROOKES, M., LAKHANI, D., FITZPATRICK, R., DAWSON, J. *et al.* (1994) 'Regular Partners and Risky Behaviour: Why Do Gay Men Have Unprotected Intercourse?', *AIDS Care*, 6, pp. 331–41.

MCMANUS, T. and MCEVOY, M. (1987) 'Some Aspects of Male Homosexual Behaviour in the UK: A Preliminary Study', *British Journal of Sexual Medicine*, 20, pp. 110–20.

OFF PINK PUBLISHING (1988) *Bisexual Lives*, London, Off Pink Publishing.

PUBLIC HEALTH LABORATORY SERVICE WORKING GROUP (1990) 'Acquired Immune Deficiency Syndrome in England and Wales to End 1993, Projections Using Data to End September 1989', Communicable Disease Report, London, PHLS Communicable Disease Surveillance Centre.

RUST, P. (1992) 'The Politics of Sexual Identity: Sexual Attraction and Behavior and Bisexual Women', *Social Problems*, 39, pp. 366–86.

SCAMBLER, G. (1984) 'Perceiving and Coping with Stigmatizing Illness', in FITZPATRICK, R., HINTON, J., NEWMAN, S., SCAMBLER, G. and THOMPSON, J. (Eds) *The Experience of Illness*, London, Tavistock Publications.

SCAMBLER, G. and HOPKINS, A. (1986) 'Being Epileptic: Coming to Terms with Stigma', *Sociology of Health and Illness*, 8, pp. 26–43.

SUNDET, J., KVALEM, I., MAGNUS, P. and BAAKKETEIG, L. (1988) 'Prevalence of Risk-Prone Sexual Behaviour in the General Population of Norway', in FLEMING, A. F. *et al.* (Eds) *The Global Impact of AIDS*, New York, Allen R. Liss.

WEATHERBURN, P. and DAVIES, P. (1993) 'Behavioural Bisexuality Among Men', in SHERR, L. (Ed.) *Heterosexual AIDS*, London, Sage.

WEATHERBURN, P., DAVIES, P., HUNT, A., COXON, A. and McMANUS, T. (1990) 'Heterosexual Behaviour in a Large Cohort of Homosexually Active Men in England and Wales', *AIDS Care*, 2, pp. 319–24.

WEEKS, J. (1987) 'Questions of Identity', in CAPLAN, P. (Ed.) *The Cultural Construction of Sexuality*, London, Tavistock Publications.

WELCH, J., PALMER, S., BANATVALA, J., BRADBEER, C. and BARLOW, D. (1986) 'Willingness of Homosexual and Bisexual Men in London to be Screened for Human Immuno-Deficiency Virus', *British Medical Journal*, 293, p. 924.

*Chapter 2*

## Bisexuality and HIV/AIDS in Canada

*Ted Myers and Dan Allman*

This chapter explores what is known about bisexuality and HIV/AIDS in Canada. It will focus primarily on research definitions, behavioural manifestations, and the political movement and organization of bisexuals in relation to HIV/AIDS. Published research, largely epidemiological, relating to the sexual behaviour of various populations since the beginning of the AIDS epidemic will be the predominant source of information. This documentation is critical because it is the only Canadian information currently available on bisexuality. While these data shed some light on the national picture as well as on regional variation, they ultimately raise more questions than answers. Scholarly reflection on sexuality in Canada and the placement of bisexuality along the continuum of human sexual relations is a discourse in its infancy. Our consideration of bisexuality in the arena of HIV/AIDS has had to take this into account.

We will first provide an overview of the sources of information on male bisexualities found in Canadian HIV/AIDS research. This will be followed by an examination of what is known from these sources regarding the proportion, distribution, social and ethnocultural characteristics, risk behaviour and the incidence of HIV infection among bisexual men. To illuminate the organization, social environment and societal responses to bisexuality, specific examples will be presented. Though many of the issues that influence the experiences of bisexuals can apply to both men and women, indeed, many of the issues may be the same, this chapter will focus exclusively on the bisexualities of men.

In terms of the number of detected infections and mortality in Canada, the HIV/AIDS epidemic has especially impacted on gay and bisexual men. Our focus on bisexual men by no means negates the experiences or realities of bisexual women, but rather reflects the patterns of HIV infection that we have witnessed in this country, and the implications this has for public health. As of October 1994, *Health Canada* reports 10,391 AIDS cases, 93.5 per cent of which are adult males. For 86 per cent of these, there is known sexual contact with a male. Eighty-nine per cent of Canada's AIDS cases have occurred in three of Canada's provinces, with 41 per cent in the Province of Ontario, 30 per cent in Québec and 18 per cent in British Columbia (Laboratory Centre for Disease Control, 1994).

### Bisexuality and HIV Research in Canada

In general, the study of sexuality in Canada remained relatively ignored until the HIV/AIDS epidemic. As in other developed countries, only in the last decade, with the realization that sexual behaviour was a primary means of transmission, has the realm of sex research begun to capture the attention of researchers and funding bodies. Unfortunately we cannot say that our review of the literature has been exhaustive. Until recently, there has been little interest in bisexual men. Few researchers have reported their results, and/or differentiated between gay and bisexual men. If a disproportionate amount of work by Myers and colleagues is reported in this paper, it is because it represents the bulk of published socio-behavioural research on gay and bisexual men and HIV in Canada.

Canadian data on bisexual men and HIV come primarily from targeted studies of men who have sex with men. Table 2.1 summarizes most of the Canadian research in which some attempt has been made to measure or define the proportion of the study population that is bisexual.[1] This research may be roughly categorized into three types: general population surveys, studies of gay and bisexual men, and studies of other populations considered to be at risk for HIV infection, such as injecting drug users, prisoners and street youth.

In Canadian studies related to HIV, the proportion of bisexual men differs depending on the definition, method of study and study population. Ornstein's (1989) random telephone survey of *AIDS in Canada* found that the proportion of male adults in the general population who reported sexual activity (previous five years) with both male and female partners was 0.9 per cent. In *The Canada Youth and AIDS Study*, 1 per cent of male college and university students and 1 per cent of male high school dropouts reported that they were bisexual (King *et al.*, 1991). A companion study found that 4 per cent of male street youth reported a bisexual orientation (Radford *et al.*, 1991).

A report on a cohort of 249 men who had sex with an HIV infected male showed that 32 per cent had sexual activity with both men and women in the eight-year period prior to data collection (between 1978 when the virus was probably present in the population and the date of recruitment in 1985) (Coates *et al.*, 1988; Calzavara *et al.*, 1991). *Men's Survey '90* (The Toronto Men's Survey) and the *Canadian Survey of Gay and Bisexual Men and HIV Infection* (The National Men's Survey) recruited men through gay-identified bars, bathhouses and, in the case of the latter, community dances. These studies found that 48 per cent of men and 54 per cent of men respectively reported sexual activity with both a man and a women in their lifetime (Myers *et al.*, 1991; Myers *et al.*, 1993a).

Interestingly, these studies of men who have sex with men have found that the proportion of the study population that report current bisexuality is fairly consistent, at about 13 per cent (definition based on reported sexual

*Table 2.1 Canadian HIV Studies that Classified Male Bisexuality*

| Source | Study Population (Recruitment) | Location | Sampling | Definition | % Bisexual Experience Lifetime | % Currently Bisexual |
|---|---|---|---|---|---|---|
| Calzavara et al., 1991 | Sexual contacts of HIV +ve men | Toronto | 249 G & B men | Sexual activity since 1978 | 32.0 | 13.3 |
| Myers et al., 1992 | Educational cohort | Toronto | 612 G & B men | Sexual activity last 5 years | 22.7 | 6.7 |
| Myers et al., 1991 | Bar and bathhouse, dance patrons | Toronto | 1,295 G & B men | Sexual activity last year | 48.3 | 13.3 |
| Myers et al., 1993a | Bar, bathhouse and dance patrons | Canada | 4,803 G & B men | Sexual activity last year<br>Sexual identity | 53.9 | 13.3<br>14.6 |
| Godin et al., 1993 | Bar, snowball, classified ads | Québec | 546 G & B men | Sexual activity last year | | 11.2 |
| Ornstein, 1989 | Telephone survey – adults | Canada | 581 males | Sexual activity last 5 years | | 0.9 |
| Myers et al., 1993b | Aboriginals living on reserves | Ontario (11 communities) | 333 males | Sexual activity lifetime<br>Sexual partner last year | 4.1 | 2.0 |
| Myers and Clement, 1994 | College students | Toronto | 707 males | Sexual activity last year | | 1.1 |

*Table 2.1* Continued

| Source | Study Population (Recruitment) | Location | Sampling | Definition | % Bisexual Experience Lifetime | % Currently Bisexual |
|---|---|---|---|---|---|---|
| King *et al.*, 1991; Radford *et al.*, 1991 | Youth | Canada | 391 street youth 596 dropouts 1,763 college | Sexual identity | 4.0 1.0 1.0 | |
| Read *et al.*, 1993 | Street youth | Toronto | 493 males | Sexual identity | 5.3 | |
| Millson *et al.*, 1995a | IDU programme evaluation | Toronto | 500 males | Sexual identity | | 5.6 |
| Millson *et al.*, 1995b | IDUs WHO collaborative study | Toronto | 809 males IDUs Non-treatment | Sexual identity | | 6.6 |
| Hankins *et al.*, 1994a | IDUs attending needle exchange | Montréal | 1,408 (M&F) | Sexual activity last 7 days | | 17.4 (M&F) |
| Hankins *et al.*, 1994b | Inmates in medium security institutions | Montréal | 971 male | Lifetime sexual activity Sexual activity 6 month pre-incarceration | 12.9 | 2.2 |

IDUs – Injecting drug users; G – Gay men; B – Bisexual men; M&F – Males and females.

activity with both a man and a woman in the last year). Lower proportions were found in the larger metropolitan areas of Vancouver and Toronto than in smaller communities, with the exception of Montréal, where a higher proportion was found. A parallel study, *Entre Hommes*, conducted in the province of Québec found that overall, 11 per cent of the study population reported current bisexuality (Godin *et al.*, 1993).

Canadian studies of men who have sex with men that have measured bisexuality have been primarily centred in the provinces of Ontario and Québec. These two provinces represent 65 per cent of the Canadian population. The National Men's Survey attempted an across-country comparison. Because of the varying sizes of Canada's gay communities, sampling by province was not possible. Consequently, it was necessary to stratify on a regional or metropolitan area basis. The data from The National Men's Survey show considerable regional variation in the lifetime sexual experience of the study population. Reports of sexual activity with both men and women ranged from a low of 35.2 per cent in the province of Québec to a high of 58.8 per cent in smaller communities in British Columbia, the Prairies, and Ontario.

Two studies of injecting drug users (IDUs), one an arm of the World Health Organization's Multicentre Study of Drug Injecting and HIV Infection, indicated that approximately 6 per cent of each of 500 and 809 male IDUs reported a current bisexual orientation (Millson *et al.*, 1995a, 1995b). In addition, Hankins *et al.* (1994a) reported that 17 per cent of 1,408 IDUs indicated sexual activity with both a man and a woman in the last seven days.[2]

Finally, 13 per cent of 971 male inmates in three medium security correctional institutions in Québec reported sexual activity with both a man and a woman in their lifetime, while 2 per cent reported themselves to be currently bisexual (defined as sexual activity with both a man and a woman in the six months prior to incarceration) (Hankins *et al.*, 1994b).

## What Is Known about Bisexuality from Canadian Research

There are no published reports in Canada in which any extensive attempt has been made to describe the characteristics of bisexual men and to distinguish these from homosexual or heterosexual men. To address this gap in part, an additional analysis of data from The Toronto Men's Survey was performed. Comparisons were made of three groups of men who have sex with men: those who reported sex with both men and women in the last year (currently bisexual), those who reported previous heterosexual experiences yet currently only had sex with men (gay – previous heterosexual) and those who, within their lifetime, indicated that they only had sex with men (gay lifetime).

Current bisexuals were younger than men identified as gay or gay but with previous heterosexual experience. Twenty-two per cent of the current bisexual group reported that they were less than 25 years of age compared with approximately 9 per cent in the other two groups. At the same time, the current bisexual group was less likely to be in a steady relationship with a man (24 per cent) compared to 34 per cent of the gay men group and 44 per cent of the gay group with previous heterosexual experience. It was hypothesized that there would be ethnoracial differences between these three groups of men who had sex with men. In fact no significant difference was found. This may reflect a bias created by a recruitment that focused on bars and bathhouses within the organized gay community, as well as a research method that relied on a fairly high degree of English literacy. The venues in which these three groups of men socialize and seek sexual partners also vary. In general, a greater proportion of bisexual men were recruited through bathhouses than through gay bars or community dances. The Toronto Men's Survey showed that 65 per cent of the currently bisexual group were recruited through bathhouses compared to less than 50 per cent for each of the other two groups.

Though these data begin to provide some basic understanding of Canadian bisexual men, they are not comprehensive and may not necessarily reflect the current situation. For example, in the last several years there has been a major development in the commercial bar scene in the City of Toronto with the emergence of a number of alternative venues and clubs which serve ethnocultural groups of men, specifically latinos. We suggest that in Canada bisexuality may be more common in men from this population. Certainly this has been the finding in much of the Latin American literature (Lumsden, 1991).

### Sexual Behaviour and Risk

While for the most part the risk behaviours of Canadian bisexual men have not been examined, The Toronto Men's Survey did include questions on eleven sexual activities that men may have engaged in during the past three

*Table 2.2 Sexual Behaviour of Respondents by Sexual Orientation*

|  | Gay Lifetime | | Gay – Previous Heterosexual | | Currently Bisexual | |
|---|---|---|---|---|---|---|
| Sexual Activity | N | % | N | % | N | % |
| No sexual activity | 34 | (11.0) | 8 | (3.5) | 11 | (13.3) |
| No anal sexual activity | 95 | (30.8) | 53 | (23.5) | 22 | (26.5) |
| Anal intercourse (protected) | 126 | (40.9) | 114 | (50.4) | 39 | (46.9) |
| Anal intercourse (unprotected) | 53 | (17.2) | 51 | (22.6) | 11 | (13.3) |

*Source: Men's Survey '90* (Toronto Men's Survey), (Myers *et al.*, 1991).

months. When recoded into a four-category variable reflecting level of risk (i.e. no sex, no anal intercourse, protected anal intercourse and unprotected anal intercourse), significant differences were found between the three subgroups of men, as shown in Table 2.2.

Currently bisexual men (13.3 per cent) and gay men (11.0 per cent) were more likely to report no sexual activity than gay men with previous heterosexual experience (3.5 per cent). The latter group were more likely to report an episode of unprotected anal sex (22.6 per cent) than were either gay men (17.2 per cent) or currently bisexual men (13.3 per cent). The bisexual men also reported having fewer male sexual partners in the last year (33.7 per cent reported ten or more sexual partners) than either gay men (47.1 per cent) or gay men with previous heterosexual experience (54.9 per cent).

### Location and Residence of Bisexuals

Extracted from The National Men's Survey, Table 2.3 shows these same three groups described above distributed across the seven sampling regions by which the country was stratified for the purpose of analysis: British Columbia and the Prairies excluding metropolitan Vancouver (VCR), Vancouver (BCP), metropolitan Toronto (TOR), Ontario excluding Toronto (ONT), metropolitan Montréal (MTL), Québec excluding metropolitan Montréal (QUE), and the Atlantic Region (ATL). Two of the sampling strata were predominantly francophone (MTL and QUE). The remaining strata were anglophone. The large sample size (4,803) ensures that the variation in proportions is meaningful.

*Table 2.3 Variation in Sexual Orientation (Behaviourally Defined) across Canada by Sampling Strata* (Total N = 4,803)

| | STRATA | | | | | | | |
|---|---|---|---|---|---|---|---|---|
| | VCR % | BCP % | TOR % | ONT % | MTL % | QUE % | ATL % | TOTAL % |
| Sexual Orientation | | | | | | | | |
| Gay | 38.4 | 38.8 | 43.1 | 39.2 | 49.9 | 62.7 | 42.9 | 43.9 |
| Current bisexual | 11.5 | 16.4 | 10.2 | 14.2 | 14.8 | 11.4 | 13.0 | 13.3 |
| Gay (previous heterosexual) | 46.5 | 42.4 | 44.8 | 44.6 | 33.5 | 23.8 | 41.3 | 40.6 |
| Other | 3.5 | 2.4 | 2.0 | 2.0 | 1.8 | 2.1 | 2.7 | 2.2 |
| (N) | (593) | (612) | (601) | (616) | (493) | (450) | (593) | (3,958) |

*Source: The Canadian Survey of Gay and Bisexual Men and HIV Infection: Men's Survey* (Myers *et al.*, 1993a).

The lowest proportion of bisexual men was found within the two English-speaking, metropolitan strata of Vancouver and Toronto. This trend was reversed in the province of Québec, including metropolitan Montréal. It has been suggested that unique differences between French and English Canada in terms of patterns of socializing, language, socialization to sexuality, and religion may account for the differences in these proportions of bisexual men. Certainly, the patterns of socializing in the francophone and anglophone gay communities differ. For example, the city of Montréal has many more bathhouses than other cities in the country.

### AIDS Hotline – An Exploratory Study

The scarcity of information on bisexual men in Canada is such that in order to develop a protocol for a future study, the authors, with the assistance of the Ontario Provincial AIDS hotline, conducted a brief feasibility study in the spring of 1994 to assess the application of the telephone as a device to recruit and interview men who have sex with both men and women. During a two-week period, callers to the hotline who volunteered that they had sex with both men and women were asked if they would agree to answer a number of questions. Almost all agreed. Sixty-one per cent of the bisexual callers were from outside of the metropolitan Toronto area.

### Relationship Status and Disclosure of Bisexuality

Forty-four per cent of the men who called the hotline were in a primary relationship with a female with occasional contact with male partner(s), 22 per cent indicated that they were in frequent contact with a variety of male and female partners, and 11 per cent indicated either that they were in a primary relationship with a male but had occasional sexual contact with females, or that they were in a dual relationship with both a man and a woman. Approximately one-third of the men who called the hotline reported that they had disclosed their bisexuality to both male and female partners, one-third of the men disclosed their bisexuality to male partners only, and 20 per cent disclosed to female partners only.

### Ways of Meeting Sexual Partners

Few of the callers to the hotline indicated that they met their sexual partners in bars or bathhouses. Rather, 41 per cent indicated that introductions by way of their social networks (not necessarily bisexual networks) were the predominant form of meeting male sexual partners, followed by encounters with partners through parks, washrooms, and automobile parking areas (24 per cent). An additional 24 per cent indicated they met their male sexual contacts through classified advertisements.

### Personal Classified Advertisements – An Exploratory Study

Allman (1994) content-analysed a systematic sample (1 in 10) of three years of voice and personal classified advertisements placed in prominent Canadian gay media. Advertisements (N = 649) were coded for the advertiser's sexual orientation, socio-demographic characteristics, the type of relationship or exchange desired, and the risk level of the requested activity as defined in the Canadian AIDS Society's *Safer Sex Guidelines* (1994). Frequently much of this information was not manifest within the text of the advertisement. Only 'codeable' advertisements that specified relevant information were included in this analysis.

Generally self-identified bisexual men were younger. Twenty-four per cent of bisexual men were below the age of 25 compared to 10 per cent of gay-identified men, while only 15 per cent of bisexual men were over the age of 40 compared to 30 per cent of gay men. There was little variation in ethnicity. Over 80 per cent of both bisexual and gay-identified men were caucasian. Sixty per cent of advertisements placed by gay-identified men requested a permanent, monogamous or long-term relationship compared to 16 per cent of those placed by bisexually identified men; while 84 per cent of advertisements placed by bisexual men requested casual sexual activity compared to 40 per cent of the advertisements placed by gay men.

In terms of risk, there was a trend for self-identified bisexual men to specify or request riskier sexual activities such as insertive and receptive anal sex. Seventy-four per cent of bisexual men specified sexual activity with some element of risk compared to 60 per cent of gay-identified men. This reflects a different pattern of risk from that found in Canadian venue-based studies, which may be because the two mediums – print and telephone – attract men of different sexual orientations or identifications. Only 7 per cent of print advertisements were placed by men who were bisexually identified, though this same group placed over 70 per cent of the voice advertisements.

### HIV Antibody Testing and HIV Infection among Bisexuals

Canadian data on HIV antibody testing among bisexual men are limited. In 1990, The Toronto Men's Survey showed bisexual men were less likely to have been tested for HIV antibodies than gay men or than gay men with previous heterosexual experience (42 per cent compared to 56 per cent in the other two groups). However, in 1991, The National Men's Survey demonstrated that an almost equal proportion of bisexual men had been tested for HIV as had gay men (60 per cent). The survey also showed the self-reported rate of HIV infection among the currently bisexual group (7 per cent) was slightly more than half that reported by the gay men or the gay men with previous heterosexual experience (12 per cent).

In addition to the studies described above, data have been made available from HIV antibody testing programmes. In the province of Ontario there are three formats for HIV antibody testing: anonymous, non-nominal and nominal. For the period January 1992 to June 1993, 10 per cent of men who tested anonymously were defined on the basis of sexual activity as bisexual compared with 1 per cent of men tested non-nominally and 0.4 per cent of men who tested nominally (Ontario Ministry of Health, 1994).

True estimates of the incidence of the HIV antibody in the Canadian population are not available. In fact the best estimates of Canadian HIV seroprevalence are derived from studies that focus on specific subgroups such as pregnant women, street youth and IDUs. Bisexuals have not been the target of such studies. In addition, there are only a limited number of studies that report on the seroprevalence of gay and bisexual men, and they do so without making the distinction between those men who are gay and those who are bisexual (Schechter *et al.*, 1987; Coates *et al.*, 1988). The scarcity of seroprevalence studies of gay and bisexual men is indicative of their controversial nature. In Canada, two reasons in particular have been used by community groups and AIDS activists to oppose seroprevalence studies. One is disagreement about the effects of such studies on the population, and the other concerns the generalizability of the results as it is not possible to determine the size of the base population on which to calculate prevalence rates.

In the Ontario voluntary HIV antibody testing programme, the seroprevalence rate among men who have sex with both men and women is lower for men testing in the anonymous programme (3.2 per cent) compared to men testing non-nominally or nominally (4.8 per cent and 5.2 per cent respectively). This is generally lower than for those men who had sex with men only with rates in the same testing modes being 6.0 per cent, 7.9 per cent and 5.6 per cent respectively (Ontario Ministry of Health, 1994).

The Ontario Ministry of Health Laboratory reports that between August and October 1993, 10 per cent of all known seroconversions involved bisexual men. Among bisexuals who were tested, 3.5 per cent were HIV antibody positive compared to 7.4 per cent of men who only reported sex with men. At the same time, 40 per cent of all positive tests of the bisexual group were seroconversions compared to only 17 per cent of the other groups. The British Columbia Centre for Disease Control report on seropositivity among street-involved persons in Vancouver (1988–92) reflects an overall rate of infection among bisexuals of 7.2 per cent compared to 16.1 per cent among homosexual men (Rekart, 1993).

Overall, Canadian research has failed to capture detail on the bisexual male and HIV/AIDS, even though information may be paramount in terms of understanding transmission of the virus. In spite of the fact that transmission of HIV from bisexual men to women is a primary concern, no attempts have been made to explore the extent to which this is happening. While the authors sense an increasing interest in bisexuality on the part of the Canadian HIV research community, this is not reflected chronologically in the research (see Table 2.1). Despite the flaws that the research reported in this chapter present, the data do provide a baseline for future research.

## The Conceptualization of Bisexuality in Canadian Research

The conceptualization of bisexuality in the fourteen Canadian studies described in this paper varies little. Essentially, two definitions have been used, one based on behaviour and the other on self-reported identity. The behavioural definitions fall primarily into two temporal dimensions – lifetime sexual experience with women and men, and sexual behaviour in the last year.

An analysis of data from The National Men's Survey comparing respondents on the basis of their behaviourally defined sexual orientation and their self-reported sexual identity reflects moderate agreement between the two definitions with 62 per cent of those whose current behaviour was bisexual (sex with men and with women in the last year) self-identifying as bisexual. An additional 31 per cent identified as gay, and 3 per cent as heterosexual. For those classified as behaviourally gay (sex with men only), and gay with previous heterosexual experience, agreement with sexual identity was greater, with 98 per cent and 88 per cent respectively indicating that they were gay or homosexual.

That behavioural definitions have been dominant in AIDS research reflects the emphasis on risk found in epidemiological thought. HIV risk has seldom been measured along a continuum. The way bisexual behaviour has been described provides us with a very limited understanding of bisexuality. It does not permit distinctions to be made between groups or individuals, and may not reflect how Canadian bisexuals perceive their own sexuality.

### Sexual Communities

In modern societies we have come to define communities beyond geographical or political boundaries and view them as communities formed around common purposes, experiences, goals and objectives. To understand the variation in the proportions of bisexuals represented in the above studies and the forms of bisexuality requires some understanding of the organization of sexuality in Canadian society. Prior to describing Canada's social and public health response towards the bisexual in relation to HIV/AIDS, we will briefly reflect on some of the interaction between the gay and bisexual communities, as well as some of the reactions of the larger society. Whether or not a bisexual community exists may be the basis for debate. There is recent reference by organized bisexuals to a Canadian 'bisexual community' although this is generally seen as a future scenario (*OBN News*, July/August 1993).

## Bisexual Networks, Organizations and Communities

It is unclear what proportion of the country's bisexuals operate within or identify with organizations such as the Ontario Bisexual Network (OBN). Many bisexual men and much of their sexual activity remain hidden. In some communities anecdotal accounts surface of individuals who provide an opportunity for bisexuals to connect or to be introduced. Theoretically these meetings are generally organized on a very informal basis. It is a phenomenon that is not well understood, and not at all researched. According to Graydon (1994) these men:

> create a network of contacts and informal sex clubs where men meet. Some informal sex clubs may be managed by one person, a kind of gate keeper, who possesses a method for contacting all players, while individual players are able only to contact him. The gate keeper arranges and hosts evenings for sex, matching up various individuals. Informal clubs may exist for weeks, perhaps while a spouse is away, or evolve to continue for years. It is not unusual that gate keepers are gay men who have made contacts with [bisexual men] over the years and who possess a place to host events.

In larger cities such networks may become more structured and organized with newsletters containing editorials, letters, articles, information and other opportunities for exchange. For example, the OBN describes itself as:

> a group formed to enable contact among bisexual people in Ontario, and to help them undertake activities of interest. At present, these activities include: a mailing list, a newsletter, support group meetings, social activities, a political action group, education of others, information sharing, and safe sexuality information. The network's only mandate is to bring people together. (OBN Meeting, 2 August 1990 as referenced in *OBN News*, May 1991)

The uniqueness of this type of organization distinguishes it from gay and lesbian groups. The OBN claims to have no overall philosophy, culture, set of beliefs or any characteristics to which one must conform, nor is the organization formed around any political agenda. Further, these groups hold a clear opposition to consensus decision-making, believing that such a model is outdated and oppressive (*OBN News*, July/August 1993). A possible movement towards organization and community development is reflected through some of the questions raised by the OBN. For example:

- Should anyone create a 'Bisexual Movement'?
- Could the idea of a movement in itself confine the bisexual action in time?
- Is anything restricted frôm the movement doomed to inertia, stagnation?
- How can this movement be liberating and for whom?

(*OBN News*, May 1991)

Questions such as these were part of the agenda for discussion at the first annual general meeting of bisexual community groups in Ontario, held in 1993.

### Gay and Lesbian Communities: Structure and Politics

Compared to Canadian bisexual communities, the organization and structure of the gay and lesbian community is much more expansive. The evolution of organized gay communities, and their political philosophies, have had an impact on bisexual community development. Among the critiques made by some gay activists in response to the increased visibility of bisexuals are the ideas that bisexuals are 'fence sitters', unable to choose between homosexuality and heterosexuality, or that bisexuals are 'confused', and their activity with both men and women is simply part of the difficult process of coming out. Some have even insinuated that bisexuals are 'piggy-backing' on gay and lesbian activism; that they wish to appropriate all the political and social advances attained by the gay movement, while maintaining the inherent freedoms and privileges of a heterosexist and homophobic society.

Overall, the political agenda of lesbian and gay communities has been more clearly defined and open, influenced in part by the strong identification that these communities have fostered. Perhaps it is because of the difficulties that many gay and lesbian organizations have had in establishing and securing gay-positive communities, as well as the need to maintain a distinction between 'straight' and 'queer' politics, that bisexuals have been excluded from the membership. For example, in one major metropolitan area, a community-funded counselling centre for lesbians and gay men preserves a policy that permits bisexuals to receive service but not to provide the same or to be a board member of the organization. Even though some of Canada's boldest opponents of racism, classism and ableism have been lesbian and gay communities, the policies, actions and opinions of some of these same communities in response to bisexuals can be labelled nothing less than biphobic.

Slowly, however, long-standing Canadian gay and lesbian organizations are beginning to change their stance, and we are currently witnessing a greater acceptance of bisexuality. This is evident in the actions of some community organizations, who have recently altered their names to include the term 'bisexual', though whether this reflects an actual change in the politics and mission statements of these groups, or is simply a semantic alteration for public relations, has yet to be determined.

## HIV Education and Bisexualities

In the early stages of the HIV epidemic the primary concern of public health officials was prevention. Until this point Canadian public health prevention and disease control initiatives had generally relied upon legislation and traditional control methods such as contact tracing. The arrival of AIDS coincided with a trend towards a 'new public health', one which embraced the principles of health promotion. Such a model favoured the provision of information and resources to individuals in order to enable and empower them to achieve and maintain their own health. Combined with this new public health paradigm was the realization that traditional models of prevention and response were not feasible or practical. In many cases an individual's contacts or sex partners would be anonymous and/or multiple. The case of bisexual men further confounded the process. Here there was the added issue of informing wives who may not have known of their husbands' activities.

Since the inception of the epidemic and the identification of unprotected anal and vaginal intercourse as major routes of HIV transmission, there has been an awareness of the risks to which Canadian bisexual men may be putting themselves and others. In addition to those they face in terms of their own health, their behaviour may entail even more risk due to their sexual activities with both men and women. From the beginning, transmission from bisexual men to their potentially unsuspecting female partners has been a concern. Some of the early incidents of HIV infection in Canadian women were cases where sexual activity with a male bisexual was identified as a risk factor. Yet, in spite of this, much of the preventive educational material aimed at transmission has referred to gay and bisexual men as a homogenous group. Early interventions applicable to bisexual men were really focused on homosexuals. This response was typical of both public health officials and community-based AIDS service organizations. HIV prevention campaigns generally avoided explicit mention of bisexual behaviour or the sexual activity of one individual with partners of both sexes. Instead efforts developed by AIDS service organizations emphasized peer group support and community building. Further, any images or messages that made reference to bisexuality did so within the context of gay identity.

In Ontario, the first educational print materials dealing with transmission facts were produced in 1983 and though the fine print did refer to bisexual men, the predominant slogan, catch phrase and sound bite was 'Gay Sex and AIDS'. By 1985, safer sex campaigns became more focused on specific messages dealing with oral and anal sex, with additional targeting to groups such as men involved in sadomasochism, and the hearing-impaired. Male bisexuals were not targeted until 1987.

Educational initiatives aimed at bisexuals have not been extensively distributed throughout the country. For the most part, public health agencies have chosen not to deal specifically with bisexual or even homosexual issues, and are often accused of being generally homophobic for their way of tackling these issues. In Toronto, the Department of Public Health became the first Canadian agency of its kind to develop an AIDS Operational Plan. The plan acknowledged bisexuality and aimed 'to provide support for risk reduction programmes for specific target groups such as drug users, prostitutes, homosexual and bisexual men and individuals with multiple sex partners' (City of Toronto, 1987).

### A Media Intervention for Bisexuals: A Case Example

Though public health response has been generally tentative, one daring educational initiative was created by the Ontario Ministry of Health. In 1990 the Ministry, on the advice of the Ministry's advisory committee recognizing the need for an educational campaign directed at bisexual men, developed a television campaign directed at five sub-populations: gay men, young women, families, IDUs and bisexual men. The process involved in the creation of the bisexual commercial included four objectives: (1) to make bisexual men aware of the risk of contracting AIDS; (2) to encourage responsible behaviour towards both male and female partners in order to protect them from HIV infection; (3) to encourage bisexual men to talk to their partners, especially female partners; and (4) to make female partners of bisexual men aware that they themselves were at risk. Certainly this was not an easy venture. Difficulties were first encountered because of the lack of research. There were no data on this group and no clear understanding about what messages might best motivate behaviour change. Second, it was conceptually difficult to know how best to typify the bisexual man and then to locate representative individuals to participate in focus groups. Ultimately the process involved the recruitment of two groups of men who currently were having sex with men, one made up of gay fathers who recently had been involved in marriages and who had children, and another comprised of men still in relationships with women.

The main goal of these focus groups was to find out what would motivate bisexual men to change their behaviour. According to participants, the answer was neither disclosure of same-sex activity to the spouse, nor the idea of self-protection. Rather, the strongest motivational factor was concern for one's family. This insight formed the basis of the first paid television advertisement of its kind in Canada. It portrayed a bisexual man returning home after a sexual encounter with a man, and expressing anxiety for not having used a condom, and concern over what this might mean for his spouse and family.

Night. Inside a car. Male driver, 30, looks into the car mirror.

> We didn't use a condom . . . He didn't want to . . .
> I should know better. What if I get AIDS?
> I could give it to Marie . . . wreck my family.

Announcer: If you have unprotected sex – even once – with a man . . . or a woman, you're risking everything. Cut the risk. Use a condom. Take charge . . . take care.

(Ontario Ministry of Health, 1992)

Though government officials and consultants developed the advertisements, approval by politicians was required. All five of the targeted population advertisements were tested for public reaction prior to wide media release, but the bisexual one also was subjected to an additional round of testing. Feedback from phone interviews in a field test of the advertisement found that 92 per cent of those who had seen the advertisement could recall some of its content, and approximately 75 per cent were left with a positive impression. Only 12 per cent of the people surveyed reacted negatively. Some people were opposed to a message that appeared to condone 'infidelity', but the evaluation concluded that the general public recognized a need for the advertisement. First shown in 1992, it continues to air today. Meanwhile the Ministry of Health is providing resources to a variety of ethnocultural groups to develop targeted campaigns. In consultation with their communities, the Chinese, Portuguese, Polish, South Asian, Caribbean and Spanish have chosen to focus at least part of their television campaigns on bisexual men.

### The Barriers, Challenges and Priorities for Research on Bisexualities in Canada

As indicated earlier in this chapter, HIV/AIDS has elevated human sexuality issues within the Canadian research community by increasing the number of persons interested in conducting research into human sexuality, and by making national and provincial funds available for such research. This chapter illustrates the limited extent to which initiatives have dealt with bisexuality. While research efforts have focused on some vital populations, for the most part the field has been dominated by biomedical and epidemiological research models, methods and criteria (National AIDS Secretariat, 1994).

HIV/AIDS in many ways has reshaped the way research is carried out. Firstly, we have seen a blending of many of the traditional disciplines. Among epidemiologists there is increased recognition of the importance of behaviour in order to understand where the epidemic is going (Chin, 1994). Boulton (1994) has emphasized some of the challenges in this area. She has noted that many of the behaviours thought to transmit HIV are private and difficult to investigate, and many of the people considered to be at high risk of HIV infection are among the least accessible to social research.

Evidence of the evolution – and need for further reshaping of the way research is carried out in Canada – is reflected in a working document prepared for Phase II of Canada's National AIDS Strategy. In the statement of principles developed for this discussion document, the importance of consultation and collaboration between researchers and community is emphasized (National AIDS Secretariat, 1994). While the principle of community-based involvement may be important to the study of bisexualities, there are logistical barriers to such an approach due to the lack of organization and the hidden nature of the population (Myers and Allman, 1995). Unlike many other marginalized minority and cultural groups, bisexuals are more likely to be scattered and not geographically grouped or centred. The potential for the development and mobilization of a bisexual community would seem to be low – particularly for the heterosexually identified man who has sex with men.

While in general it would appear easier to undertake research in Canada on male bisexual communities and bisexual activity than it would be in other, less developed countries, this is not necessarily the case. Preparatory and developmental work is required of Canadian society in general as one of the major barriers to research has been the country's response to bisexuality. Canadian society has marginalized bisexuals and has responded to them with even greater intolerance, suspicion and confusion than to other groups of men who have sex with men. This is seen in both the response by the lesbian and gay community and by society at large. The sophistication and community development of the gay and lesbian communities, and their stances on bisexuality, have meant that many of these men have chosen to remain hidden beneath heterosexual and homosexual identities. In the years since the emergence of AIDS, police have continued to arrest men, many of whom are bisexual, in public places such as washrooms where sex is known to occur (*Globe and Mail*, 5 July 1993; *Globe and Mail*, 3 September 1993). While HIV/AIDS educators have for some time seen the need for outreach in the locations where men meet and engage in sexual activity such as parks and washrooms, only now are we beginning to see attempts to contact these men in their milieu. Organizations who choose to initiate programmes discover that extensive effort is required. The issue is twofold. While educators wish to tread carefully so as not to scare away these men who have sex with men, they do wish to guarantee the safety and security of outreach personnel and volunteers.

Techniques to locate these men for educational and prevention purposes and to recruit these men for research may be similar. In some communities, the success of initiatives may not rest solely with the social organization of bisexual men but also with the police, public health officials and the judicial system. These authorities may have policies that scrutinize places where bisexual men may be seeking sexual partners, and therefore limit outreach and contact with these men. As suggested earlier by Allman's analysis (1994), some of the more traditional methods of contacting and finding sex partners may be replaced by the modern technologies of telephone networks and computer bulletin boards.

In the absence of a strong foundation of research into bisexualities and HIV/AIDS in Canada, the research agenda remains open. Following Chu *et al.* (1992) we can identify a number of critical issues for study in Canada. Risk behaviour, as discussed in this chapter, has been too closely defined in the context of gay sex. Often the assumption is that bisexual men do not take precautions and do not disclose their sexual activity to female partners. This has never been empirically confirmed. In addition greater understanding is needed of the social and sexual networks of bisexuals. Some preliminary qualitative work within ethnocultural groups has shown there are important differences to explore (Adrien *et al.*, 1994). While researchers have found some difference in homosexual and bisexual activity between English and French language groups in Canada, we do not understand why this is so, or whether similar differences exist for other language groups.

## Canadian Sexuality and Bisexuality in Perspective

Canada is one of the largest of the world's developed countries, with a land mass of almost 10 million square kilometres. In contrast the population is relatively small with only 27 million inhabitants. Canadian sexualities would appear to reflect an environment characterized by a vast and varied terrain, a mitigating climate and a population of fluctuating density. Historically this country's reputation as 'the new world' has implied a land of opportunity, and as a result Canada continues to attract new immigrants from every country in the world. Rather than promote a melting-pot society, our multicultural policies celebrate differences between communities. Though this culture has evolved side by side in a symbiotic relationship with the United States, we believe there remains a unique Canadian identity.

The racial heritages and ethnocultural backgrounds of the original settlers and the subsequent displacement of First Nation or aboriginal people have impacted on our perceptions of sexuality (Bullock, 1995). As well, the social and political organization of the ten provinces and two territories and Canada's role in international politics bear upon what is known and understood about sexuality and bisexuality in the country. Canada has been described as a 'vertical mosaic' (Porter, 1969), a multitude of institutionally complete ethnic communities that permit wide variation in community association – and, we would add, sexual identification. That some men from these communities would engage in sexual activity with both men and women is not in question. What we do not know is how the sexual norms of each of these communities may interact within a Canadian context.

It is the authors' contention that bisexuality has long been ignored in Canada's HIV/AIDS prevention, education and research efforts. Ultimately, it has not been possible in this chapter to explore all of the themes that 'Canadian bisexualities' may suggest. Hard data on bisexuality have not been readily available and in deference, a wide variety of sources have been collected in order to uncover what, for the most part, has been an untouched subject.

## Notes

1 Some of the percentages in this table have not been previously reported and were provided by the researchers specifically for the purpose of this chapter.
2 This figure combines male and female injecting drug users.

## References

ADRIEN, A., GODIN, G., CAPPON, P., MANSON-SINGER, S., MATICKA-TYNDALE, E. and WILLIAMS, D. (1994) *Many Voices: HIV/AIDS in the Context of Culture. Ethnocultural Communities Facing AIDS: A National Study*, Ottawa, National AIDS Clearinghouse.

ALLMAN, D. (1994) 'Personal Classified Advertisements of Men Seeking Sex with Men: Trends in Representations of Risk Behaviour, 1980–1994', presentation at the Fourth Annual Canadian Conference on HIV/AIDS Research, Toronto, Ontario.

BOULTON, M. (1994) 'The Methodological Imagination', in BOULTON, M. (Ed.) *Challenge and Innovation: Methodological Advances in Social Research on HIV/AIDS*, London, Taylor & Francis.

BULLOCK, S. L. (1995) 'The Perceptions of Sex among First Nations People Living On-Reserve in Ontario', unpublished Masters thesis, University of Toronto.

CALZAVARA, L., COATES, R., JOHNSON, K., READ, S., FAREWELL, V., FANNING, M., SHEPHERD, F. and MACFADDEN, D. (1991) 'Sexual Behaviour Changes in a Cohort of Male Sexual Contacts of Men with HIV Disease: A Three Year Overview', *Canadian Journal of Public Health*, 82, 3, pp. 150–6.

CANADIAN AIDS SOCIETY (1994) *Safer Sex Guidelines: Healthy Sexuality and HIV. A Resource Guide for Educators and Counsellors*, Ottawa, Canadian AIDS Society.

CHIN, J. (1994) 'HIV/AIDS Surveillance: How Accurate and/or Useful Are the Numbers?', presentation at the Fourth Annual Canadian Conference on HIV/AIDS Research, Toronto, Ontario.

CHU, S. Y., PETERMAN, T. A., DOLL, L. S., BUEHLER, J. W. and CURRAN, J. W. (1992) 'AIDS in Bisexual Men in the United States: Epidemiology and

Transmission to Women', *American Journal of Public Health*, 82, 2, pp. 220–4.

CITY OF TORONTO, DEPARTMENT OF PUBLIC HEALTH (1987) *AIDS Operational Plan Implementation Proposal 1987–1989*, Toronto, Ontario.

COATES, R., CALZAVARA, L., READ, S., FANNING, M., SHEPHERD, F., KLEIN, M., JOHNSON, J. and SOSKOLNE, C. (1988) 'Risk Factors for HIV Infection in Male Sexual Contacts of Men with AIDS or an AIDS-Related Condition', *American Journal of Epidemiology*, 128, 4, pp. 729–39.

*GLOBE AND MAIL* (1993a) Toronto, Ontario, 5 July.

*GLOBE AND MAIL* (1993b) Toronto, Ontario, 3 September.

GODIN, G., CARSLEY, J., MORRISON, K. and BRADET, R. (1993) *Entre hommes 91–92: Les comportements sexuelles et l'environment social des hommes ayant des relations sexuelles avec d'autres hommes*, Québec, COCQ sida.

GRAYDON, M. (1994) 'Divided Loyalties – Reaching Straight Men who Have Sex with Men: Safer Sex Outreach to Heterosexually Identified Men who Have Sex with Men', paper at 8th Annual British Columbia HIV/AIDS Conference, November.

HANKINS, C., GENDRON, S. and TRAN, T. (1994a) 'CACTUS – Montréal: Profile comportemental de la clientèle et prévalence de l'infection par le VIH', Rapport 5, December.

HANKINS, C., GENDRON, S. and TRAN, T. (1994b) *Risk Factors for HIV Infection in Inmates of Medium Security Correctional Institutions*, Montréal, Centre for AIDS Studies.

KING, A., BEAZLEY, R. P., WARREN, W. K., HANKINS, C. A., ROBERTSON, A. S. and RADFORD, J. L. (1991) *Canadian Youth and AIDS Study*, Kingston, Social Program Evaluation Group, Queen's University.

LABORATORY CENTRE for DISEASE CONTROL, Division of HIV/AIDS Epidemiology, Bureau of Communicable Disease Epidemiology, Health Canada (1994) *Surveillance Update: AIDS in Canada*, Ottawa, October.

LUMSDEN, I. (1991) *Homosexuality: Society and the State in Mexico*, Toronto, Canadian Gay Archives.

MILLSON, P., MYERS, T., RANKIN, J., MCLAUGHLIN, B., MAJOR, C., MINDELL, W., COATES, R., RIGBY, J. and STRATHDEE, S. (1995a) 'Prevalence of Human Immunodeficiency Virus and Associated Risk Behaviour in Injection Users in Toronto', *Canadian Journal of Public Health*, 86, 3/4.

MILLSON, P., MYERS, T., RANKIN, J., FEARON, M. and MAJOR, C. (1995b) 'WHO Multicentre Study of Drug Injecting and HIV Infection', Toronto Centre, Final Report of NHRDP Grant 6606-4694-AIDS.

MYERS, T. and ALLMAN, D. (1995) 'The HIV/AIDS Epidemic and Community-Research Partnerships in Canada', in READY, M. and TAGGART, M. E. (Eds) *'Une Approche heuristique et multidisciplinaire. Réflexions et stratégies pour les professionels de la santé'*, Montréal, Morin Ltée.

MYERS, T. and CLEMENT, C. (1994) 'Condom Use and Attitudes among Heterosexual College Students', *Canadian Journal of Public Health*, 85, 1, pp. 51–5.

MYERS, T., LOCKER, D., ORR, K. and JACKSON, E. (1991) *Men's Survey '90 – AIDS: Knowledge, Attitudes, Behaviours. A Study of Gay and Bisexual Men in Toronto*, Toronto, AIDS Committee of Toronto.

MYERS, T., TUDIVER, F., KURTZ, R., JACKSON, E., ORR, K., ROWE, C. and BULLOCK, S. (1992) 'The Talking Sex Project: Description of the Study Population and Correlates of Unsafe Sexual Practices at Baseline', *Canadian Journal of Public Health*, 83, 1, pp. 47–52.

MYERS, T., GODIN, G., CALZAVARA, L., LAMBERT, J. and LOCKER, D. (1993a) *Canadian Survey of Gay and Bisexual Men and HIV Infection: Men's Survey*, Ottawa, Canadian AIDS Society.

MYERS, T., CALZAVARA, L., COCKERILL, R. and MARSHALL, V. (1993b) *Ontario First Nations AIDS and Health Lifestyle Survey*, Toronto, University of Toronto.

NATIONAL AIDS SECRETARIAT (1994) *Towards a National HIV/AIDS Research Planning Process: A Discussion Paper*, Ottawa, National AIDS Secretariat.

*OBN NEWS* (1991) Toronto, Ontario, May.

*OBN NEWS* (1993) Toronto, Ontario, July/August.

ONTARIO MINISTRY OF HEALTH (1992) *HIV/AIDS Education in Ontario: From Information to Behaviour Change, the Evolution of AIDS Television Advertising*, Toronto, Ontario Ministry of Health.

ONTARIO MINISTRY OF HEALTH (1994) *Anonymous HIV Testing Evaluation – January 1992 to June 1993*, Toronto, AIDS Bureau.

ORNSTEIN, M. D. (1989) *AIDS in Canada*, Toronto, University of Toronto Press.

PORTER, J. (1969) *The Vertical Mosaic: An Analysis of Social Class and Power in Canada*, Toronto, University of Toronto Press.

RADFORD, J., KING, A. and WARREN, W. (1991) *Street Youth and AIDS*, Kingston, Social Program Evaluation Group, Queen's University.

READ, S., DeMATTEO, D., BOCK, B., COATES, R., GOLDBERG, E., KING, S., MAJOR, C., McLAUGHLIN, B., MILLSON, M. and O'SHAUGHNESSY, M. (1993) *HIV Prevalence in Toronto Street Youths*, Toronto, Hospital for Sick Children.

REKART, M. (1993) 'Trends in HIV Seroprevalence among Street-Involved Persons in Vancouver, Canada (1988–1992)', presentation at the IXth International Conference on AIDS, Berlin.

SCHECHTER, M. T., BOYKO, W. J., CRAIB, K. J. P., McLEOD, A., WILLOUGHBY, B., DOUGLAS, B., CONSTANCE, P. and O'SHAUGHNESSY, M. (1987) 'Effects of Long-Term Seropositivity to Human Immunodeficiency Virus in a Cohort of Homosexual Men', *AIDS*, 1, pp. 77–82.

## Chapter 3

# Not Gay, Not Bisexual, but Polymorphously Sexually Active: Male Bisexuality and AIDS in Australia

*June Crawford, Susan Kippax and Garrett Prestage*

Australia is one of a very few countries where HIV infection and AIDS continue to be highly concentrated among men who engage in male-to-male sex. In this chapter, we will examine Australian research on men who engage in both homosexual and heterosexual activity. On the whole, these men do not think of themselves as 'bisexual', although some of them may do so. It is difficult to decide on an appropriate descriptive term for such men – elsewhere we have sometimes referred to them as 'men who have sex with both men and women' – a very cumbersome solution to the problem. Dowsett (1994) writes of them as 'homosexually active', although this too is problematic when he writes of 'gay and other homosexually active men' since we would then need to refer to them as 'homosexually and heterosexually active'. Since this book is about 'bisexualities', we shall use the term 'bisexually active' for the sake of brevity, whilst acknowledging the problematic status of the term, particularly as it tends to gloss over the fact that sexual practices are either homosexual or heterosexual and are not (except in some rare instances) bisexual. The same is true for sexual encounters.

By the end of September 1994, there had been 5,324 reported cases of AIDS in Australia, of whom 3,826 (72 per cent) have died. Ninety-six per cent of these reported cases of AIDS had occurred in males, and 1 per cent among people under 20 years of age. The patterning of AIDS has been remarkably stable over the years, with male-to-male sexual transmission accounting for 83 per cent of cases of AIDS, and male-to-male sexual contact and injecting drug use accounting for a further 4 per cent. (Note that the category 'male-to-male sexual contact and injecting drug use' refers to an ambiguity with respect to whether transmission was through male-to-male sex or through injecting drug use.)

Percentage figures for HIV diagnoses are similar to those for AIDS, though in recent years the decline in actual numbers of new diagnoses attributed to male-to-male sexual contact and male-to-male sexual contact with injecting drug use has seen a slight decrease in percentage terms (from 83 per cent to 81 per cent and from 4 per cent to 3 per cent respectively). Australia also has a very small proportion of cases of HIV transmission through injecting drug use, with this category (5 per cent of HIV diagnoses) representing a smaller percentage than that for heterosexual contact (7 per cent).

Heterosexual transmission of HIV has remained stable for a number of years. Each year since 1990 there have been around 130 new diagnoses of HIV infection attributed to heterosexual transmission. Since the beginning of the epidemic there have been 819 such diagnoses, 499 men and 320 women. So far there is no evidence that HIV infection through heterosexual transmission is increasing (National Centre for HIV Epidemiology and Clinical Research, 1995). As Dowsett (1994, p. 5) points out:

> This patterning of HIV infection and AIDS suggests two explana-
> tions: (1) that efforts to date in Australia to contain HIV within the
> gay community have been largely effective, through the combination
> of specific and continuous prevention work in the gay communities
> and general population prevention education, or (2) that the *policing
> of sexual boundaries* in Australian sexual culture is sufficiently rigorous
> so as to hinder the effective transmission of HIV from the population
> first and hardest hit by the epidemic, i.e. gay men. It is most probable
> that a combination of these two is closest to the mark.

This chapter interrogates Australian research on bisexually active men from this perspective. First, it assesses what is known about such men when compared with exclusively homosexual men. Where possible, we also compare those who are not socially or culturally attached to a gay community with those who are. We include in our examination: demographic characteristics, relationship status, 'sexual identity', the nature of the contexts in which bisexual men engage in male-to-male sex, including relationship status, places where male sexual partners are sought and places where male-to-male sex is practised; safety of male-to-male sex; and, where possible, information about heterosexual sexual practice.

Research from the United Kingdom (Boulton *et al.*, 1992) suggests that there are three significant contexts of bisexual activity, namely embedded in a heterosexual context, embedded in a gay context, and embedded in a bisexual context. A tripartite typology of bisexuality has also been suggested by the Australian research of Buchbinder and Waddell (1992) to be dealt with below. The research to be reported in some detail in this chapter enables a fairly clear distinction to be made between men whose activities appear to be embedded in a heterosexual context and those where they are embedded in a gay context. Little information is available about a distinctly bisexual context. The nature of the epidemic in Australia and also the nature of the samples on which research has been based makes the distinction between non-gay-community-attached bisexually active men and those who are gay-community-attached a relevant and important one. In this chapter we argue that as well as a social separation between these two groups, male-to-male sex has different meanings for these two groups of men.

In order to explore the meanings of male-to-male sex for bisexually active men, we explore data from two large surveys of bisexually active men and two more focused qualitative studies. The evidence suggests that bisexually active men, particularly those who are separated socially from gay communities, distance themselves emotionally from their male partners. A consideration of the variety of meanings of male-to-male sex together with information about the contexts in which it is practised support the notion of boundaries which are 'policed'. Both gay-community-attached bisexually active men and those who are not gay-community-attached for different reasons do not appear to constitute a large 'threat' to the general population in Australia at this stage.

### Early Australian Research

In the mid to late 1980s, there were a number of Australian studies providing information about the sexual practices of bisexually active men in the context of the HIV epidemic. Three early studies were primarily concerned with men who were recruited through gay community sources, and hence attached to gay community. These studies, namely the Melbourne University study (Campbell *et al.*, 1988; Burgess *et al.*, 1990), the SAPA study (Kippax *et al.*, 1993), and the distinctively named 'Operation Vampire' (Frazer *et al.*, 1988) included limited information about bisexually active men.

Taken as a whole, these studies showed that around 10 per cent of men recruited largely from gay community sources were bisexually active, defined as reporting sex with a female partner around the time of the survey, usually within the previous six months. When these men's practices were compared with those of the remainder of the group, few differences in sexual practice or knowledge of HIV transmission were found (Campbell *et al.*, 1988; Kippax *et al.*, 1993). Bisexually active men were likely to have lower levels of social and cultural engagement in gay community, and slightly less likely to be using condoms consistently than those who did not have sex with women. Levels of condom use in vaginal and/or anal sex with women were quite low (Kippax *et al.*, 1993).

Further research on samples with large proportions of bisexually active men was carried out in the late 1980s by Bennett *et al.* (1989). They recruited men from bars, sex shops and 'beats' – public parks and toilets where men can find male sexual partners for occasional sexual encounters. In a follow-up study (Prestage and Crawford, unpublished report) another sample of fifty-eight men were interviewed at beats and a further seventy-one men were interviewed by telephone after responding to advertisements in personal columns of local newspapers. In this second study, men who were gay-identified or socially attached to a gay community were excluded.

When comparing the results of the studies of Bennett (now Prestage) with those recruited mainly from gay communities, it is clear that bisexually active men who were not attached to a gay community were much more likely to be married, less likely to have a regular male partner, and more likely to self-identify as heterosexual. They were very unlikely to have disclosed their male-to-male sexual activity to friends or family. One finding from the second study was that, particularly for the men interviewed by telephone, there was a preference for receptive anal intercourse. Around 55 per cent engaged in receptive but not insertive anal intercourse. It was not possible from these data to determine what proportion of these men used condoms consistently, though 47 per cent used condoms at least some of the time.

Other notable differences in sexual practice were that only 60 per cent of non-gay-attached bisexually active men engaged in kissing with their male partners, whereas this practice was almost universal (89 per cent) in a sample of predominantly gay men (Connell and Kippax, 1990; Kippax *et al.*, 1993). Qualitative data from the second Prestage study, and from a qualitative study where men were recruited for telephone interviews using the same strategy (O'Reilly, 1991), indicated that the meanings of male-to-male sex were different for these men. They tended to use terms like 'just fooling around', 'kinky', or 'different' to refer to male-to-male sexual activity. Prestage and Crawford (unpublished report) reported evidence showing that the telephone sample had some of the attributes of 'sexual adventurers'. When asked what sexual activities they would be interested to try (or had tried), they were interested in a great many, including those sometimes regarded as esoteric, such as S-M/bondage, and voyeurism.

In general, bisexually active men who were not gay-community-attached had low levels of interest in 'soft' sexual practices with male partners, such as kissing, massage, and sensuous touching, and low interest in spending the whole night with a male partner. They were likely to name anal intercourse, particularly receptive anal intercourse, as the most physically satisfying male-to-male sexual practice and also as the most emotionally satisfying. This last finding, however, has not been replicated in more recent research using larger samples (see below).

The above studies were all carried out in the late 1980s and the sizes of the samples of bisexually active men in these studies were quite small, ranging from fifty-four to seventy-one. This research confirmed that there are two groups of bisexually active men, namely those who are attached to a gay community and those who are not. This was largely, though not entirely, a function of the ways in which the samples were recruited.

### More Recent Studies

More recently, two Australian studies have obtained information from fairly large samples of bisexually active men. In 1992, the Commonwealth Government commissioned a telephone survey of men who have sex with men in Australia, known as Project Male-Call (Kippax *et al.*, 1994). This resulted in a national sample of 2,583 men, of whom 761 were bisexually active. In 1992–3, another telephone survey was carried out in New South Wales in which 698 men were interviewed, of whom 372 had had sex with a woman within the previous six months. This project was called the BANGAR project (Bisexual and Non-Gay Attached Research) and aimed to interview men from Sydney and two rural centres who were not attached to a gay community (Hood *et al.*, 1994). Two further qualitative studies have also been carried out based on smaller samples. Bartos *et al.* (1993) interviewed ninety-seven men in Victoria, around half of whom were bisexually active. These men were non-gay-community-attached. Buchbinder and Waddell (1992) also obtained interview data from seventy-eight bisexually active men in Western Australia.

The remainder of this chapter examines findings from these more recent studies with respect to bisexually active men. The Male-Call sample was recruited using a wide range of strategies, most of those interviewed had responded to advertisements in either the gay or mainstream press (including suburban newspapers). Men in the BANGAR study were recruited mainly through advertisements in personal columns of suburban newspapers, usually published weekly, and delivered free of charge to most residences.

We first examine data from the two large surveys (Project Male-Call and BANGAR). It should be pointed out that there has been more research done in Australia focused on bisexually active men who are non-gay-community-attached than on those who are attached to gay communities. This is particularly true in the case of qualitative research.

### Characteristics of Bisexually Active Men in the Surveys

It was found in Project Male-Call, which sampled 'men who have sex with men', that there were essentially two populations of men, one which had very little social or political attachment to a gay community (non-gay-community-attached) and one with varying levels of such attachment (Kippax *et al.*, 1994). Of bisexually active men, 60 per cent were non-gay-community-attached and 40 per cent were gay-community-attached.[1]

Bisexually active men differed from exclusively homosexual men in a number of ways. Apart from obvious characteristics such as living with a female sex partner, to have had children or to have been married, there were few demographic differences found in Project Male-Call between bisexually active men and exclusively homosexual men. Differences found were that bisexually active men were significantly less likely to be tertiary educated, and more likely to have occupations in categories of trade and manual occupations (Kippax *et al.*, 1994; Rodden *et al.*, 1994). Levels of HIV infection were low. Only 1.6 per cent of bisexually active men knew themselves to be HIV positive, compared with 8.8 per cent of exclusively homosexual men. Fewer bisexually active men had been tested, however (57.2 per cent as opposed to 81.6 per cent).

In the BANGAR study, urban areas generally regarded as being 'working-class' and one rural area were targeted. Men were excluded if they were assessed on the basis of a series of questions as being socially or politically attached to a gay community. In the BANGAR study, bisexually active men were younger than the non-gay-community-attached bisexually active men in Project Male-Call, with significantly more men in the under 20 age group (9.8 per cent compared with 5.9 per cent), and they were significantly more likely to have only low levels of education. A slightly higher proportion of them were engaged in trade and manual occupations. Over 40 per cent were married or living with a female sexual partner.

### Patterns of Sexual Practice

#### With Men

In terms of sexual practice with male partners, findings from earlier studies which were confirmed included relatively low levels of kissing (both deep and dry) and sensuous touching with male partners, and some suggestion of higher levels of engagement in 'esoteric' practices. Bisexually active men reported significantly higher levels of fisting than did exclusively homosexual men, though in absolute terms the percentage engaging in this practice was low (under 10 per cent) (Kippax *et al.*, 1994).

In the more recent research (Hood *et al.*, 1994; Kippax *et al.*, 1994) there is no suggestion that receptive anal intercourse is more frequent among bisexually active men as found in earlier research. Indeed, in the BANGAR study, men who said they 'preferred' sex with women, and were likely to identify as heterosexual rather than bisexual, were least likely to engage in anal intercourse with male partners, particularly unprotected anal intercourse (Hood *et al.*, 1994). No significant differences were found between the two groups of bisexually active men (those who were non-gay-community-attached and those who were gay-community-attached) with respect to the percentages engaging in anal sex with male partners, nor with respect to consistent use of condoms for anal intercourse with male partners.

#### With Women

In Project Male-Call, men were asked about sexual practices with women in the past six months. Practices which were almost universal (over 90 per cent) included sensuous touching, kissing (both wet or deep and dry), and vaginal finger-fucking (Kippax *et al.*, 1994). This may be contrasted with the low levels of engagement in similar 'soft' practices with men. Vaginal intercourse was also engaged in by over 90 per cent of bisexually active men, and there was a surprisingly high level of anal intercourse with women (32 per cent), by

*49*

*Table 3.1  Condom Use in Sexual Practices with Women for Two Groups of Bisexually Active Men*

| | Non-gay-community-attached bisexually active men (N = 459) | | | Gay-community-attached bisexually active men (N = 302) | | | Total (N = 761) | | |
|---|---|---|---|---|---|---|---|---|---|
| | Total N | N | % | Total N | N | % | Total N | N | % |
| (a) Casual partners | | | | | | | | | |
| Vaginal intercourse with ejaculation** | 183 | 86 | 47.0 | 171 | 103 | 60.2 | 354 | 189 | 53.4 |
| Vaginal intercourse without ejaculation*** | 88 | 22 | 25.0 | 69 | 29 | 42.0 | 157 | 51 | 32.5 |
| Anal intercourse with ejaculation*** | 63 | 30 | 47.6 | 57 | 42 | 73.7 | 120 | 72 | 60.0 |
| Anal intercourse without ejaculation*** | 36 | 8 | 22.2 | 36 | 20 | 55.6 | 72 | 28 | 38.9 |
| (b) Regular partners | | | | | | | | | |
| Vaginal intercourse with ejaculation*** | 336 | 45 | 13.4 | 154 | 39 | 25.3 | 491 | 84 | 17.1 |
| Vaginal intercourse without ejaculation*** | 133 | 13 | 9.8 | 68 | 15 | 22.1 | 201 | 28 | 13.9 |
| Anal intercourse with ejaculation** | 107 | 27 | 25.2 | 58 | 21 | 36.2 | 165 | 48 | 29.1 |
| Anal intercourse without ejaculation | 55 | 8 | 14.5 | 35 | 6 | 17.1 | 90 | 14 | 15.6 |

*Notes:* Total N is the number engaging in the practice; N and percentages are those using condoms 'always'.

Levels of significance for $\chi^2$ test
***p < 0.001
**p < 0.01

comparison for example with the results of the British general population survey which found only around 7 per cent of heterosexuals had engaged in anal intercourse in the previous year (Wellings *et al.*, 1994).

Levels of condom use for either vaginal or anal intercourse with female partners were low (see Table 3.1). Figures for condom use in heterosexual practice are comparable with those of the general population in Australia. It will be noted that bisexually active men who were gay-community-attached were significantly more likely to use condoms 'always' in sex with female partners than those who were non-gay-community-attached.

### Interpersonal Context of Male-to-Male Sex

In Project Male-Call, bisexually active men were very likely to have either occasional male partners or no regular male partners (65 per cent). When compared with exclusively homosexual men, bisexually active men in Project Male-Call had fewer male partners in the previous six months and in a lifetime. Thirteen per cent of bisexually active men had had no male-to-male sex in the previous six months (Kippax *et al.*, 1994). Bisexually active men who were non-gay-community-attached had significantly fewer male partners in the previous six months and in a lifetime than those who were attached to a gay community.

The overwhelming impression gained from studies of bisexually active men is of the diversity of interpersonal contexts in which male-to-male sex takes place. As researchers, we have not always given sufficient recognition to the wide diversity of interpersonal relationships that exist among homosexually active men, even among those who are attached to a gay community. We have sometimes tended to use the terms 'regular' and 'casual' relationships as if the categories 'regular' and 'casual' are relatively straightforward. In discussing bisexually active men in particular, the 'regular'/ 'casual' distinction is one which may need to be reconsidered. Since many bisexually active men have a primary relationship which is heterosexual, they tend to regard all male-to-male sexual activity as 'casual'. Some of these partners, however, are people who are well known and of long-standing acquaintance or friendship, for example an old school friend or a relative. Even though the sex itself is 'casual', and occurs on occasions when the partners meet haphazardly, and somewhat infrequently, the relationship between the partners is not what one would ordinarily term 'casual'. On the other hand, many male-to-male sexual encounters of bisexually active men are anonymous, often non-verbal, such as those that take place in beats or, as one respondent described it, on 'a moving train'.

When asked where they go to find casual male partners, bisexually active men most frequently responded in the categories of from among friends, at beats, and in another town. There appears to be a bimodal pattern, not necessarily mutually exclusive, of finding casual partners on the one hand in the course of social interaction such as at private parties and from among friends, where sex is in a sense a by-product of social interaction, and on the other hand finding casual partners in settings designed primarily for a sexual encounter such as at beats and to some extent through advertisements. Although there were statistically significant differences between non-gay-community-attached and gay-community-attached bisexually active men with respect to the proportions responding in the various categories, these are in general explained by the finding that in almost all categories, gay-community-attached men were more likely than non-gay-community-attached men to say that they sought casual male partners in that setting (see Table 3.2).

While both groups are more likely to say that they find casual male partners from among friends and at beats, it is very likely that the 'friends' and the location of the beats are different. Differences in geographic location as well as (sub)cultural differences between the groups suggest that the beats where non-gay-community-attached men find partners are removed from the

*Table 3.2 Places Where Two Groups of Bisexually Active Men Seek Casual Male Partners and Percentage of those with Casual Male Partners who Responded that they Seek Such Partners in Each Setting*

| Source | Non-gay-community-attached bisexually active men (N = 357) | Gay-community-attached-bisexually active men (N = 255) | Total (N = 612) |
|---|---|---|---|
| | % | % | % |
| Gay bars*** | 21.6 | 50.2 | 33.5 |
| Straight bars*** | 21.0 | 38.4 | 28.3 |
| Saunas | 31.7 | 39.2 | 34.7 |
| Discos/dances*** | 14.3 | 46.7 | 27.8 |
| Parties/friends*** | 33.3 | 71.4 | 49.1 |
| Beats | 40.3 | 45.9 | 43.4 |
| Work | 6.7 | 12.9 | 9.4 |
| Sex on premises | 16.8 | 22.4 | 21.0 |
| Another town*** | 33.9 | 53.3 | 42.1 |
| Sex cinemas | 18.5 | 18.8 | 18.7 |
| Street prostitutes | 3.9 | 6.7 | 5.1 |
| Brothels | 16.5 | 13.3 | 15.2 |
| Gym*** | 13.2 | 26.3 | 18.7 |
| Pool/beach*** | 28.9 | 51.0 | 38.2 |
| Advertisements in gay press | 25.8 | 36.9 | 30.4 |
| Advertisements in mainstream press*** | 25.1 | 25.1 | 25.1 |

Levels of significance for $\chi^2$ test
***p < 0.001
**p < 0.01

centres of gay culture which many of the gay-community-attached men would use. Differences in 'beat cultures' have been noted by Davis *et al.* (1991).

## Situational Context of Male-to-Male Sex

There is considerable overlap between the interpersonal and the social/situational context in which male-to-male sex takes place. Sex at a beat is very likely to be impersonal, for example. Bisexually active men in Project Male-Call were most likely (55 per cent) to have had sex with a casual partner at the home of the partner ('his place') and/or at the home of the respondent (37.3 per cent). Other places were beats (27.5 per cent), saunas (17 per cent), sex on premises of venues (11.2 per cent) or elsewhere (29.9 per cent) (Crawford *et al.*, 1993). These figures are very similar to those found for the bisexually active men in the BANGAR study.

### Meanings of Male-to-Male Sex

If it is the case that, for bisexually active men, male-to-male sex takes place in contexts separated from gay community, then it is also likely that male-to-male sex has meanings which differ from those of exclusively homosexual men. Meanings will also differ for non-gay-community-attached bisexually active men and for those who are gay-community-attached. Information about such meanings is obtainable somewhat indirectly from survey studies such as Project Male-Call, slightly more directly from the small amount of qualitative information gathered from the sample in the BANGAR study, in some detail from the work of Buchbinder and Waddell (1992), and more directly from the in-depth work described in Bartos *et al.* (1993).

In Project Male-Call, respondents were asked which sexual practices with men they found to be most emotionally satisfying. Whereas over 50 per cent of the exclusively homosexual men responded in the categories of kissing, touching and massage, fewer than 20 per cent of the bisexually active men did so. On the other hand, 16 per cent of the bisexually active men responded 'nothing is emotionally satisfying, it's only physical' (only 4 per cent of exclusively homosexual men responded in this way). Bisexually active men were more likely to nominate oral-genital sex as most emotionally satisfying (25 per cent), and around 20 per cent of both groups nominated anal intercourse.

In the BANGAR study, men were asked what they liked about having sex with other men. Most frequently mentioned were oral sex (around 50 per cent), anal sex (around 25 per cent) and 'partner's body' (23 per cent) – in this question the categories were not mutually exclusive. A very small proportion (10 per cent) named kissing and/or sensuous touching (cuddling). When asked about sexual practice on the last occasion on which they had male-to-male sex, only 9.3 per cent of the men in the BANGAR study said that they engaged in kissing and/or sensuous touching.

What can be made of these findings? First, it is clear that bisexually active men (particularly those in a primary on-going relationship with a female partner) are unlikely to engage in 'soft' practices of kissing and/or sensuous touching with male sexual partners. On the other hand, they almost universally engage in such practices with female partners. They also differ greatly from exclusively homosexual men in the extent to which they regard these practices with men as emotionally satisfying, and a sizeable minority (again, this is even more sizeable for non-gay-community-attached bisexually active men) stated spontaneously that 'nothing is emotionally satisfying' about sex with men.

The work of Bartos *et al.* (1993) can help in suggesting ways of interpreting these data. The research was based on interview material with bisexually active men (and other non-gay-community-attached homosexually active men). From the bisexually active men, a picture emerges which helps to explain the finding that bisexually active men often do not engage in kissing (and possibly other 'soft practices') with their male partners. One such man said:

> I have been doing it with men for almost 24 years. Men suck me off. I don't touch the men I have sex with. I don't kiss them. I love my wife and want to stay with her, so I don't touch or do anything which may create a closeness or intimacy with these men. I am also not really gay. Gay sex is something that I do 2–3 times a week. It amounts to so little of my time. If you were to add up the time I spend looking for and having sex with men it would total 1–2 hours weekly. The rest of the time I am heterosexual, married, a family man. (quoted in Bartos *et al.* (1993), p. 29)

Another said:

> I'm not gay. If I was gay, I would kiss the men I have sex with. I never kiss men. I only kiss women I go to bed with. If I was gay I would kiss men, and I don't. (quoted in Bartos *et al.* (1993), p. 29)

The bisexually active men in the Bartos *et al.* (1993) study, as opposed to those who were exclusively homosexual, were inclined: (1) to avoid intimacy with their male sexual partners; (2) to be conscious of the need to protect their female partners by using condoms for anal sex (and even sometimes for oral-genital sex), and (3) to maintain a distance from the gay community. Some men explained their male-to-male sex as a result of a compelling and 'unusually strong sex drive' (Bartos *et al.*, 1993, p. 43).

In all three studies, bisexually active men who were not attached to a gay community appeared to accept their own sexual behaviour, that is, it was not problematic for them. Although concerned not to disclose their male-to-male sexual activity, they, like the first man quoted above, managed it to their own satisfaction and discussed it in fairly matter-of-fact terms. For example, 'It's not important to me. I do it with men on occasions. . . . It's no one's business what I do on my odd afternoon off' (Bartos *et al.*, 1993, p. 27), and 'Every now and then, I do it with a man, that's all'.

For such men, sexual practice with men is not seen as central to their lives and certainly not central to their sense of who they are. They deliberately distance themselves emotionally from their male partners, they relegate their practice of male-to-male sex and the contexts in which it takes place to the periphery of their lives. What is central for them is their primary identity as a husband, father, family man. Sex with men is detached both emotionally and socially from this primary identity. Bartos *et al.* (1993, p. 43) reported that '[some] men expressed the view that they would prefer not to have sex with other men, but that they had a compulsion to do so'.

Bisexually active men who are attached to a gay community also need to be considered. As already mentioned, it was found in earlier work (Campbell *et al.*, 1988; Frazer *et al.*, 1988; Burgess *et al.*, 1990; Kippax *et al.*, 1993) that around 10 per cent of primarily gay-attached samples of men had had sex with a woman in the previous six months. In Project Male-Call, (Kippax *et al.*, 1994), 40 per cent of bisexually active men were gay-community-attached. Meanings of male-to-male sex for these men are likely to be quite different. Meanings of male-to-male sex for bisexually active men who are gay-community-attached may be more similar to those of exclusively homosexual men. There is little qualitative data on which to base an assessment of meanings of male-to-male sex for bisexually active men who are attached to gay communities. The survey data regarding physically and emotionally satisfying sexual practices with men suggests that such meanings may be similar to those found for exclusively homosexual men who are attached to gay communities. It may well be that for gay men who are bisexually active, their sexual practice with men is more central to their lives, their identity as gay or homosexual or bisexual is more central to their sense of self, and what (if anything) may be problematic for these men is their sex with female partners. In one of the few in-depth studies which included a proportion of gay-community-attached bisexually active men, Buchbinder and Waddell (1992) found that the group of 'bisexual' men least likely to express positive feelings about their sexuality were those who were most 'homosexual'. The distinction we have made between the two kinds of bisexually active men may be to some extent concordant with the tripartite distinction suggested by Buchbinder and Waddell (1992) on the basis of research carried out in Western Australia. They suggest that there are three types of bisexual men, namely those who are in general sexually active with women but with occasional homosexual activity, those who are essentially homosexual but with occasional heterosexual activity, and those who engage 'impartially' in sex with either women or men. Even though this distinction appears to complicate notions of heterosexuality, homosexuality and bisexuality, and is to some extent concordant with that made by Boulton *et al.* (1992), we would argue that it is still an oversimplification. As the title of this chapter suggests, our data would support a more complex view such as that proposed earlier by Boulton and Coxon (1991), that is, that there are many and varied patterns of sexual practice and erotic desire within the broad groupings that we have considered.

### Policing the Boundaries

The nature of the HIV/AIDS epidemic in Australia, particularly the concentration of the virus in places close to centres of gay culture, makes relevant the distinction we have made between two groups of bisexually active men using a rough index of gay community attachment. We would argue that bisexually active men, whether attached to a gay community or not, do not at this stage of the epidemic in Australia represent a 'threat' of changing the nature of the epidemic at least in the short term. For those men not attached to a gay

community, their identity as essentially heterosexual and their desire to protect themselves, their partners and families from the consequences of unsafe
male-to-male sex is one reason why HIV transmission from the homosexual to
the heterosexual community on a widespread scale appears unlikely at
present. In addition to their sexual practices, the distance, both geographic
and social, of these men from gay communities makes it relatively unlikely that
they will become infected since their sexual partners are unlikely to be HIV
antibody positive. Finally, many of them engage in male-to-male sex relatively
infrequently.

These men are unlikely to cross the boundary into the gay community.
They engage in 'self-policing' of such a boundary, maintaining their emo-
tional as well as their physical distance from it. They fear being seen in gay
bars, for example, and resist the idea of seeking help or information from
AIDS Councils, which are perceived as gay organizations (Bartos *et al.*, 1993;
Hood *et al.*, 1994).

Dowsett (1994) makes the point that heterosexist notions of the relationship between emotion and intimacy for example may need to be abandoned,
but we would argue that heterosexist meanings of sexuality and sexual practice are those within which at least some bisexually active men frame their
lives. As Buchbinder and Waddell (1992) argue, the problematic fact of male
bisexuality is accounted for in two ways by both the culture and the dominant
model of masculinity. The first is consistent with a view of masculinity that is
part of the sociobiological discourse of a strong male sex drive, that is, that
male bisexuality is regarded as evidence of a potent male sexuality 'so potent
as to be effectually indifferent to the sex of the individual's partners' (p. 181).
The second view of male bisexuality is to see a bisexually active man as in fact
gay, but pretending to be heterosexual. Evidence from the studies of bisexually active men who are not gay-community-attached suggests that they deny or
do not accept the second view, though some, such as those in the Bartos *et al.*
(1993) study who felt 'compelled' to engage in male-to-male sex, would appear to share the first view.

While bisexually active men who are not attached to a gay community to
some extent police the boundary from without, there is also a policing of the
boundary from within gay communities. Bisexually active men who are attached to a gay community are reluctant to disclose their heterosexual activities to other gay men (Kippax *et al.*, 1994), and to some extent they feel less
comfortable with their 'bisexual' identity (Buchbinder and Waddell, 1992).
Buchbinder and Waddell (1992, p. 170) offer several possible explanations,
including the suggestion that 'the political dynamics of gay worlds may be
such that heterosexual activity is viewed as letting the side down'.

Bisexually active men from within gay communities are unlikely to pose a
large 'threat' because of their generally higher levels of safe sex practice with
women, and their exposure to the safe sex messages and safe sex culture of gay
communities. There is nevertheless room for improvement in these men's
levels of safe sex, with both male and female partners. More research is also

needed in order to add to an understanding of ways in which safe sex messages may be made more effective for men in this group.

### Implications for HIV Prevention: A Bridge to the General Community?

It may seem logical or rational to propose that the pattern of the HIV epidemic in Australia (and to some extent in other Western countries such as Great Britain, the United States, Canada, The Netherlands, Switzerland and Germany) dictates that bisexually active men constitute a group of particular importance in that they provide an actual or potential bridge between the homosexual (gay) and heterosexual (general) populations.

To some extent, the apparent boundaries of the epidemic in Australia conform with such a notion, but we would argue that although the epidemic is concentrated among the gay communities it is not confined to them. That is, although, as we have argued, the boundaries are policed, largely as a result of conscious or unconscious self-policing, they are not impermeable. The practices of bisexually active men which place them and their partners (both male and female) at risk are a potential means of transmitting the virus. The idea that bisexual men constitute a 'group' which can be viewed as a 'bridge', however, sets up a false notion that a military-style defensive operation can be concentrated at a single (metaphorical) location such as a bridgehead.

What our analysis shows is that although there is a degree of separation, geographic, subcultural, and psychological, between many bisexually active men and the gay communities, such separation is by no means absolute. Bisexually active men are to be found on both sides of the boundaries, and some undoubtedly cross them either wittingly or unwittingly when they engage in male-to-male sex. So far, the maintenance of fairly high levels of safe sex practice within the gay communities and the practices of bisexually active men both within and outside of gay communities will not result in rapid increases in HIV infection outside of those communities. Nevertheless the potential for such increases remains, and the danger posed to the female partners of bisexually active men is a real one, in view of the comparatively unsafe nature of bisexually active men's practices with their female partners.

Thus it is important to maintain policies which continue to support, reinforce, and increase the practice of safe sex within gay communities. Policies and programmes for bisexually active men are also needed, and they need to be designed in the light of the complex and sometimes contradictory information regarding the diversity of meanings of male-to-male sex. For bisexually active men both within and outside of gay communities, the now well established findings that sexual identity and sexual practice do not necessarily correspond is a challenge that must be met by any such programmes.

**Note**

1 We have used the notion of gay community attachment to distinguish two groups of bisexually active men. In Project Male-Call (Kippax *et al.*, 1994), this was formalized by using a scale developed previously (Kippax *et al.*, 1992, 1993) to measure social engagement in gay community. This scale consisted of items such as number of gay male friends, and social activities engaged in with such gay male friends. In the BANGAR study (Hood *et al.*, 1994), a set of questions designed to assess overall attachment to gay community was used to exclude potential interviewees. The study by Bartos *et al.* (1993) relied to some extent on service providers to identify men who were not attached to a gay community, and augmented the sample so obtained by the use of newspaper advertisements similar to those used in the BANGAR study.

**References**

BARTOS, M., McLEOD, J. and NOTT, P. (1993) *Meanings of Sex Between Men* [A study conducted by the Australian Federation of AIDS Organizations for the Commonwealth Department of Human Services and Health], Canberra, Australian Government Publishing Service.

BENNETT, G., CHAPMAN, S. and BRAY, F. (1989) 'A Potential Source of Transmission of AIDS to the Heterosexual Populations: Bisexual Men who Frequent "Beats"', *Medical Journal of Australia*, 151, pp. 309–14.

BOULTON, M. and COXON, T. (1991) 'Bisexuality in the United Kingdom', in TIELMAN, R., CARBALLO, M. and HENDRIKS, A. (Eds) *Bisexuality and HIV/ AIDS: A Global Perspective*, New York, Prometheus.

BOULTON, M., HART, G. and FITZPATRICK, R. (1992) 'The Sexual Behaviour of Bisexual Men in Relation to HIV Transmission', *AIDS Care*, 4, 2, pp. 165–75.

BUCHBINDER, D. and WADDELL, C. (1992) 'Myth-Conceptions about Bisexual Men', *Southern Review*, 25, 2, pp. 168–84.

BURGESS, P. M., GOLLER, I. E., FINCH, S. J. and PEAD, J. (1990) *A Prospective Study of Factors Influencing HIV Infection in Homosexual and Bisexual Men: Interim Report of Findings – Stage II*, Melbourne, University of Melbourne, Department of Psychology.

CAMPBELL, I. M., BURGESS, P. M., GOLLER, I. E. and LUCAS, R. (1988) *A Prospective Study of Factors Influencing HIV Infection in Homosexual and Bisexual Men: A Report of Findings – Stage I*, Melbourne, University of Melbourne, Department of Psychology.

CONNELL, R. W. and KIPPAX, S. (1990) 'Sexuality in the AIDS Crisis: Patterns of Sexual Practice and Pleasure in a Sample of Gay and Bisexual Men', *Journal of Sex Research*, 27, 2, pp. 1–32.

CRAWFORD, J., KIPPAX, S. and DOWSETT, G. W. (1993) 'Bisexual Men and Safe Sex Practice', paper presented at the IXth International AIDS Conference, Berlin, July. Abstract No.WS-D07-1.

DAVIS, M. D., KLEMMER, U. and DOWSETT, G. W. (1991) *Bisexually Active Men and Beats: Theoretical and Educational Implications* [Report of the Bisexually Active Men's Outreach Project], Sydney, AIDS Council of New South Wales and the Macquarie University AIDS Research Unit.

DOWSETT, G. W. (1994) *Sexual Contexts and Homosexually Active Men in Australia: Revisited Considerations for a National HIV/AIDS Educational Intervention*, Canberra, Commonwealth Department of Human Services and Health, August.

FRAZER, I. H., McCAMISH, M., HAY, I. and NORTH, P. (1988) 'Influence of Human Immunodeficiency Virus Antibody Testing on Sexual Behaviour in a "High-Risk" Population in a "Low-Risk" City', *Medical Journal of Australia*, 149, pp. 365–8.

GIFFORD, S. M., MITCHELL, A., ROSENTHAL, D. and TEMPLE-SMITH, M. (1994) *STD and HIV/AIDS Education for People of Non-English Speaking Backgrounds* [Report by the Centre for the Study of Sexually Transmissible Diseases, La Trobe University, for the Commonwealth Department of Human Services and Health], Canberra, Australian Government Publishing Service.

HOOD, D., PRESTAGE, G., CRAWFORD, J., SORRELL, T. and O'REILLY, C. (1994) *Bisexual Activity and Non-Gay-Attachment Research: The BANGAR Report*, Sydney, Western Sydney Area Health Service.

KIPPAX, S., CRAWFORD, J., CONNELL, R. W., DOWSETT, G. W., WATSON, L., RODDEN, P., BAXTER, D. and BERG, R. (1992) 'The Importance of Gay Community in the Prevention of HIV Transmission: A Study of Australian Men who Have Sex with Men', in AGGLETON, P., DAVIES, P. and HART, G. (Eds) *AIDS: Rights, Risk and Reason*, London, Falmer Press.

KIPPAX, S., CONNELL, R. W., DOWSETT, G. W. and CRAWFORD, J. (1993) *Sustaining Safe Sex: Gay Communities Respond to AIDS*, London, Falmer Press.

KIPPAX, S., CRAWFORD, J., RODDEN, P. and BENTON, K. (1994) *Report on Project Male-Call: National Telephone Survey of Men Who have Sex with Men* [Report from the National Centre for HIV Social Research, Macquarie University, to the Commonwealth Department of Human Services and Health], Canberra, Australian Government Publishing Service.

McCAMISH, M., COX, S., FRAZER, I. H. and NORTH, P. (1988) 'Self-Reported Changes in Sexual Practices among Gay and Bisexual Men as a Result of AIDS Awareness in a "Low-Risk" City', paper presented at the IVth International Conference on AIDS, Stockholm, Sweden, June. Abstract No. 6536.

NATIONAL CENTRE IN HIV EPIDEMIOLOGY AND CLINICAL RESEARCH (1995) *Australian HIV Surveillance Report*, 11, 1.

O'REILLY, C. (1991) *Western Sydney Men who have Sex with Men Project*, Sydney, Western Sydney Area Health Service.

PRESTAGE, G. and CRAWFORD, J. (unpublished report) Report of the Second Sydney Beats Study, Macquarie University.

RODDEN, P., CRAWFORD, J. and KIPPAX, S. (1994) 'Project Male-Call: Class Differences in Sexual Practice', in AGGLETON, P., DAVIES, P. and HART, G. (Eds) *AIDS: Foundations for the Future*, London, Taylor & Francis.

WELLINGS, K., FIELD, J., JOHNSON, A. and WADSWORTH, J. (1994) *Sexual Behaviour in Britain: The National Survey on Sexual Attitudes and Lifestyles*, Harmondsworth, Penguin Books.

*Chapter 4*

# Bisexuality and AIDS: Results from French Quantitative Studies

*Antoine Messiah and the ACSF Group[1]*

Since the start of the AIDS epidemic in France, men with homosexual and bisexual behaviour have formed the majority of recorded cases: constituting an absolute majority until 1988, then a relative majority, the progressive fall in their share of cases reflecting an increase among other groups (Réseau National de Santé Publique, 1994). The importance of efforts to prevent HIV transmission among behaviourally homosexual and bisexual men was clear, but the effectiveness of such measures depended on an accurate understanding of the characteristics of people for whom they were developed. The absence of such understanding triggered a series of studies on the socio-demographic characteristics, opinions, attitudes, beliefs and practices of gay men, conducted mainly through the gay press (Pollak and Schiltz, 1991a; Schiltz, 1993). However, as is suggested by the use of the category term 'homo-bisexual' in French AIDS statistics (Réseau National de Santé Publique, 1994) and in behavioural reports (e.g. Pollak and Schiltz, 1991a), the world of sex was divided – for males – into two: those who had sex with men, regardless of any coexisting heterosexual activity, and those who had not. This remained the case, even after epidemiologists drew attention to the possible consequences that bisexual activity among men could have with the AIDS epidemic (Chu *et al.*, 1992; Lifson, 1992; Wood *et al.*, 1993; Krijnen *et al.*, 1994). Men having sex with both men and women offer a challenge for public health research, demanding urgent answers to the following among other questions (Messiah *et al.*, 1994, 1995): are such men easily reached by gay-oriented prevention messages; does their behaviour play an important role in the heterosexual spread of HIV; and what role does male bisexual behaviour play in maintaining the HIV epidemic among gay men? At the start of the epidemic in France, the lack of data which could help to answer, even partly, these questions was surprising.

When addressing questions of so-called 'sexual orientation' or 'sexual choice', most French quantitative studies place individuals in one of two categories: heterosexual or homosexual (Lhomond, 1993). What tended to happen, when reported sexual activity resulted in a conflicting categorization, were efforts to retain this dichotomy, with the men concerned being allocated to the more socially rejected category – homosexual – a practice for which there was no epidemiological justification, especially prior to the advent of AIDS. Thus, bisexual men virtually did not exist, either because they were categorized as homosexuals (in the 'homo/bisexual' category) or because no attention was paid to how the two different sets of activities – homosexual and heterosexual – were combined. At most, homosexual experience was mentioned in the context of studies devoted mainly to an analysis of heterosexual behaviour (e.g. Simon *et al.*, 1972; Léridon, 1989; Lagrange, 1991) or conversely, instances of heterosexual intercourse were reported as transient activities within the context of a homosexual 'coming out' (Pollak and Schiltz, 1991b). Thus, bisexuality was disregarded for years, although data elsewhere suggested that it could be a relatively common practice among men having sex with men (Schmidt *et al.*, 1989; Rogers and Turner, 1991; Smith, 1991). For these reasons it was felt that much could be gained by analysing data from population-based samples such as that in the recent French study on sexual behaviour, the Analyse des Comportements Sexuels en France (ACSF), and in paying special attention to the behavioural and socio-demographic characteristics of men having both homosexual and heterosexual activities.

## ACSF Methodology and its Limitations

The methodology used to draw the ACSF sample has been well described elsewhere (e.g. ACSF Investigators, 1992; Léridon and Bozon, 1993; Messiah and Mouret-Fourme, 1993; Spira *et al.*, 1994; Messiah *et al.*, 1996) so here we will restrict ourselves to an outline of its main characteristics and the influence sampling procedures may have had on the selection of subsamples of homosexual and bisexual men.

The ACSF survey is a large-scale population-based telephone survey. It is based on a primary random sample of 20,055 individuals, aged between 18 and 69 years and French-speaking, selected from the telephone directory between September 1991 and February 1992. These individuals participated in a fifteen-minute interview in the course of which they were asked if any of the following were true: (1) had they had intercourse with at least two different people in the previous twelve months; (2) had they had sexual intercourse with at least one person of the same gender in the previous five years; (3) had they paid or been paid for sexual intercourse in the previous five years; (4) had they used a hard or soft drug in the last year; and (5) were they born on the 4th, 17th or 20th of any month.

The 4,820 individuals who satisfied at least one of the above criteria, but did not have to specify which one(s), participated in a longer interview.[2] Overall, 2,642 men were selected, 2,547 of whom provided detailed information about their sexual activity. These included those who had had sexual intercourse with another man in the previous five years, this response option being included as one of a number of others in a single general question. Also included were men whose last homosexual intercourse had taken place more than five years ago, if one of the other criteria applied. The classification of these men as homosexual, bisexual or heterosexual took place *a posteriori*, and was based on responses to subsequent questions about the gender and the number of their partners at different periods of their life. The homosexual and bisexual men in the survey were thus selected by a random procedure, without having been questioned directly about a sexual identity that so often proves difficult or impossible to talk about overtly (Pollak and Schiltz, 1987), and which is not considered as an accurate behavioural indicator (Chu *et al.*, 1992; Wood *et al.*, 1993; Ekstrand *et al.*, 1994; Wellings *et al.*, 1994). Instead, they were categorized according to their recent sexual activity.

However, distortions affecting participation and compliance in the interview may still have arisen, and the direction of these and the degree to which they cancel each other out are unknown (Messiah and Mouret-Fourme, 1993). General population-based studies are likely to suffer from under-representation and under-reporting of stigmatized practises (Wellings *et al.*, 1994), but include men who have sex with men whether or not they identify as gay (Messiah and Mouret-Fourme, 1993; Wellings *et al.*, 1994). Thus, in spite of the expected (and observed) small subsample size, data from this study complement well findings from surveys directed specifically at male homo-bisexuals, the latter being likely to over-represent participants in the commercial gay scene, or readers of the gay press (Messiah and Mouret-Fourme, 1993; Pollak and Schiltz, 1991b).

For the statistical analysis, responses were weighted in order to take into account the complex sample design (Cochran, 1977; Lee *et al.*, 1989). Descriptive and comparative analysis was carried out using Sudaan software (Shah *et al.*, 1993).

## Defining Bisexual Activity

Since bisexual activity, which does not necessarily mean bisexual self-identification, is characterized by the coexistence of two activities that are somewhat in competition (availability for one often implies unavailability for the other), its study is strongly sensitive to the time interval over which questions about sexual behaviour are asked. Problems may also arise from how bisexual activity is defined, but will generally be related to the question of defining sexual behaviour itself (Bajos *et al.*, 1994). In the ACSF survey, interviewees were left to decide what is sexual and what is not, without referring to any particular definition; they were classified as homosexual, bisexual or heterosexual, according to the gender of their partners for the period under scrutiny. Since data on sexual behaviour are considered to be reliable provided the period of recall is not overly long (Catania *et al.*, 1990; Upchurch *et al.*, 1991), our classification was based on activity during the previous year. In specific instances, however, we also enquired further back.

## Bisexual Activity: Patterns of Mixing Sex Partner's Gender

Since the definition of bisexual activity is much a matter of defining which period of time is under scrutiny, once sexual behaviour has been defined (or, as here, left undefined), we will first examine how numbers of men defined as behaviourally bisexual are affected by choosing a given period.

Of the men interviewed, 41 per thousand declared having had at least one male sex partner in their life; among them the great majority (39.6 per thousand) had also had heterosexual experiences. Looking at shorter time intervals gives a more polarized picture. Eleven men per thousand reported bisexual activity, and a further 3 per thousand reported exclusively homosexual activity in the last five years. In the last year, 7 per thousand reported bisexual activity (later referred as 'bisexuals'), and a further 4 per thousand exclusively homosexual activity (later referred as 'homosexuals'). Thus, even when restricting the analysis to a short and recent period, bisexuality seems relatively common among men having sex with men, provided they were selected neither through the gay scene nor through the gay press. From the numbers given for each period being considered, one can quantify the relationship between the different poles of activity for each period examined.

Although bisexuals seem more frequently to have phases of heterosexuality than of homosexuality, their homosexual preference appears clearly when taking into account the relatively small number of potential homosexual partners in relation to heterosexual ones (Messiah and Mouret-Fourme, 1993). Such a preference has also been found by studies using purposive samples (Schiltz *et al.*, 1993) but could be caused by biases in sampling procedures; the ACSF survey shows that this was not the case.

Table 4.1 reports the mean number of sexual partners reported by different groups of men. Bisexual men are situated mid-way between exclusively homosexual men who have more partners, and heterosexual men who have fewer, being in many ways comparable to multi-partnered heterosexuals (two or more partners in the past year). The composition of their sexual network is balanced between male and female partners, whatever the period considered. Examining the nature of this multiple partnership, we find 31 per cent of them heterosexually multi-partnered, against 13 per cent among heterosexuals; and 28 per cent homosexually multi-partnered, against 63 per cent among exclusively homosexual men. An analysis of relationship between each type of multiple partnership reveals that they are independent (Messiah and Mouret-Fourme, 1993); each one neither favours nor prevents the other. Thus bisexuals appear to be situated mid-way between homosexuals and heterosexuals, differing from multi-partnered heterosexuals by the mixed gender composition but not by the size of their sexual network. When addressing other aspects of the sexual life of bisexuals, *multi-partnered heterosexuals are therefore likely to be the heterosexual* group of reference.

Table 4.1 Number of Sexual Partners (Means) and Socio-Demographic Characteristics (Column Percentages) of Bisexual Men Compared with Homosexual Men, Heterosexual Men with Multiple Partners, and Heterosexual Men At Large (Classification Based on Past Year's Activity).

| | Past year's activity | | | | Comparisons | | |
|---|---|---|---|---|---|---|---|
| | (1) Heterosexual n = 2359 | (2) Multi-partnered heterosexual n = 104 | (3) Bisexual n = 53 | (4) Homosexual n = 52 | 3 vs 1 | 3 vs 2 | 3 vs 4 |
| **Number of partners** | | | | | | | |
| Past five years | | | | | | | |
| Total | 2.9 | 8.7 | 7.0 | 16.2 | * | ns | * |
| Male | 0.0 | 0.0 | 3.0 | 15.4 | – | – | – |
| Female | 2.9 | 8.7 | 4.0 | 0.8 | – | – | – |
| Past year | | | | | | | |
| Total | 1.3 | 3.0 | 2.8 | 4.1 | * | ns | * |
| Male | 0.0 | 0.0 | 1.2 | 4.1 | – | – | – |
| Female | 1.3 | 3.0 | 1.5 | 0.0 | – | – | – |
| **Socio-demographic characteristics** | | | | | | | |
| Age | | | | | | | |
| 18–25 | 18 | 35 | 22 | 19 | | | |
| 26–45 | 49 | 44 | 41 | 63 | ns | ns | ns |
| 46–69 | 33 | 21 | 37 | 19 | | | |
| Living as a couple | 75 | 44 | 68 | 29 | ns | * | * |

Table 4.1 Continued

| | Past year's activity | | | | Comparisons | | |
|---|---|---|---|---|---|---|---|
| | (1) Heterosexual n = 2359 | (2) Multi-partnered heterosexual n = 104 | (3) Bisexual n = 53 | (4) Homosexual n = 52 | 3 vs 1 | 3 vs 2 | 3 vs 4 |
| Residence | | | | | | | |
| Provincial town | | | | | | | |
| ≤100,000 inhabitants | 56 | 47 | 47 | 14 | | | |
| >100,000 inhabitants | 27 | 31 | 33 | 39 | ns | ns | * |
| Paris area | 17 | 22 | 20 | 47 | | | |
| Education: high school graduate | 33 | 41 | 53 | 68 | * | ns | ns |
| Current or last occupation | | | | | | | |
| Blue-collar and farm workers | 35 | 28 | 30 | 4 | | | |
| Middle-class jobs | 40 | 36 | 24 | 43 | ns | ns | ns |
| Upper-middle-class jobs | 17 | 19 | 35 | 35 | | | |
| Never employed | 8 | 17 | 11 | 18 | | | |

*Note*: in comparisons, ns = non-significant; * p < 0.05.

### Socio-Demographic Characteristics

The age distribution of bisexual men is very similar to that of heterosexual men surveyed. It contrasts, although without significant difference, with that of both multi-partnered heterosexuals and exclusively homosexual men. The presence of numerous bisexuals in the maturer age groups indicates that bipolar activity can be maintained into later life; it contradicts a view according to which bisexuals end up by choosing between heterosexuality and homosexuality (Pollak and Schiltz, 1987, 1991b). However, it may also be that some of these bisexuals are 'authentic' homosexuals belonging to a generation on which society imposed heterosexual behaviour.

Living in couples is another similarity between bisexual and heterosexual men. Of the 68 per cent of bisexual men reporting living as a couple, 28 per cent did so as a homosexual couple and 40 per cent as a heterosexual couple. Bisexuals are as likely as multi-partnered heterosexuals to form heterosexual couples, and as likely as exclusively homosexual men to form homosexual couples. Area of residence is a third characteristic that bisexuals share with heterosexuals (the similarity being more striking with multi-partnered heterosexuals), contrasting with a Parisian concentration of homosexuals (to the detriment of small-sized provincial towns). Similar contrasts between homosexual and bisexual men were found in surveys among readers of the gay press (Schiltz *et al.*, 1993).

Educational level shows a remarkable unequal distribution: with one in two high school graduates, bisexuals occupy a half-way position between heterosexual men (lower educated) and exclusively homosexual men (higher educated). There were no clear trends in socio-economic status across groups, except for the fact that blue-collar and farm workers, equally well represented among bisexuals and heterosexuals, were markedly under-represented among exclusively homosexual men. These results reflect the difference between a random sampling survey like ACSF and surveys conducted among readers of the gay press, for which no major contrast between homosexual and bisexual men was found (Schiltz *et al.*, 1993). Thus bisexual men differ from exclusively homosexual men in numerous respects: they are more similar to heterosexual men on several socio-demographic indicators, and otherwise occupy an intermediate position between homosexual and heterosexual men.

The socio-demographic contrasts between bisexual and homosexual men can be interpreted through the light of sociological work. The under-representation of homosexual men among manual workers and farmers probably lies in the low social acceptability of overt homosexuality in these milieux (Pollak and Schiltz, 1987, 1991c), which is responsible for strategies of escape (Pollak, 1991; Pollak and Schiltz, 1991b). In order to achieve this escape, homosexual men make a higher than average investment in education, particularly in the case of individuals from working-class backgrounds (Pollak, 1982). These educational and professional itineraries are paralleled by a geographical migration to urban centres (Pollak, 1988; Pollak and Schiltz,

*Table 4.2 Bisexual Men Compared to Homosexual and Heterosexual Men with Multiple Partners (Classification Based on Past Year's Activity): Sexual Practices in Most Recent Homosexual and Heterosexual Encounters (Column Percentages)*

| Sexual practices | Last heterosexual encounter[†] | | Last homosexual encounter[†] | |
| | Multi-partnered heterosexuals n = 1027 | Bisexuals n = 36 | Bisexuals n = 36 | Homosexuals n = 51 |
|---|---|---|---|---|
| Subject masturbated by the partner | 41 | 52 | 75 | 78 |
| Partner masturbated by the subject | 65 | 69 | 77 | 88 |
| Partner's self-masturbation | 12 | 13 | 51 | 51 |
| Subject's self-masturbation | 6 | 9 | 40 | 49 |
| Subject's finger into partner's vagina | 74 | 86 | | |
| Cunnilingus | 40 | 51 | | |
| Partner's penis into subject's mouth | | | | |
| No | | | 23 | 36 |
| With condom | | | 8 | 6 |
| Without condom | | | 69 | 58 |
| Subject's penis into partner's mouth | | | | |
| No | 56 | 57 | 19 | 31 |
| With condom | 3 | 2 | 13 | 8 |
| Without condom | 41 | 41 | 67 | 61 |
| Vaginal penetration | | | | |
| No | 2 | 9 | | |
| With condom | 20 | 12 | | |
| Without condom | 78 | 79 | | |
| Insertive anal penetration | | | | |
| No | 94 | 90 | 56 | 74 |
| With condom | 1 | 1 | 17 | 14 |
| Without condom | 5 | 9 | 27 | 12 |
| Receptive anal penetration | | | | |
| No | | | 66 | 81 |
| With condom | | | 11 | 11 |
| Without condom | | | 22 | 8 |

† = no comparisons were significant.

1987, 1991b) which offer better conditions for the expression of homosexual sentiments. It is also possible, however, to imagine a reciprocal mechanism at work (Messiah and Mouret-Fourme, 1993): of the homosexual men from hostile backgrounds, only those who do succeed in escaping by means of education are actually able to live their homosexuality fully, whereas the rest are constrained by social pressure to lead a bisexual or even an exclusively heterosexual existence. Thus, some of the bisexual men could be 'authentic' homosexuals who, given their socio-demographical environment, are obliged to maintain the pretence of a heterosexual life.

### Elements of a Bisexual Repertoire

Practices during the last sexual encounter were investigated in detail (see Table 4.2). Multi-partnered respondents were questioned about their two most recent partners, who in the case of bisexuals could have been men, women or both. Thus, thirty-six of the fifty-three bisexual men described at least one homosexual encounter – to be compared to the last encounter of homosexuals (n = 51) – and thirty-six described at least one heterosexual encounter – to be compared to the last encounter of multi-partnered heterosexuals (n = 1027). No differences reached significance, probably due to small sample sizes and subsequent lack of power, but some trends are worth highlighting. Although heterosexual and homosexual practices are not to be directly compared, we presented them when possible on the same lines in Table 4.2, in order to facilitate a comparison between each repertoire.

Bisexuals were similar to heterosexuals in the frequency of almost all their practices, this being particularly marked in the case of unprotected penetrative sex. The same was not true on the homosexual side: unprotected penetrative practices were systematically more frequent among bisexuals. When specific practices could be directly compared, their frequencies were higher on the homosexual side than on the heterosexual one, suggesting a more diversified repertoire.

Thus bisexual men seem to engage in HIV-risk-related homosexual practices more frequently than homosexual men do. This is not balanced by lower risk on the heterosexual side, since they are similar to multi-partnered heterosexuals regarding the frequency of unprotected heterosexual practices. Surveys among readers of the gay press have also revealed that in France bisexuals are less likely than homosexuals to practise safer sex (Schiltz *et al.*, 1993).

### Preventive Behaviours and HIV Testing

As shown in Table 4.3, bisexual men were less likely to engage in HIV preventive behaviour than homosexual men. Although an analysis of behaviour one

Table 4.3 Bisexual Men Compared to Homosexual and Heterosexual Men with Multiple Partners (Classification Based on Past Year's Activity): Preventive Behaviours and HIV Testing (Column Percentages)

| | Past year's activity | | | Comparisons | |
|---|---|---|---|---|---|
| | (2) Multi-partnered heterosexual n = 1040 | (3) Bisexual n = 53 | (4) Homosexual n = 52 | 3 vs 2 | 3 vs 4 |
| Ever using condom during past year | 58 | 59 | 52 | ns | ns |
| Having given up penetration† | 3 | 28 | 49 | * | ns |
| Ever having had an HIV test | 33 | 35 | 66 | ns | * |
| Asking new partners to have HIV test† | 5 | 14 | 34 | ns | ns |
| Questioning partners about their sexual history† | 36 | 53 | 53 | ns | ns |
| Having sex only when in love with the partner† | 30 | 22 | 50 | ns | * |
| Having sex only with known persons† | 38 | 40 | 56 | ns | ns |
| Diversity of behaviours: average number of above behaviours in which indulging | 1.8 | 1.9 | 2.6 | ns | * |

Note: in comparisons, ns = non-significant; *p < 0.05.

† These questions were formulated as 'behavioural changes since people started talking about AIDS'.

at a time revealed few significant differences, most reported frequencies were lower among bisexuals. In order to summarize these trends, we counted the number of behaviours the subjects had engaged in: bisexuals had significantly engaged in fewer behaviours than homosexuals, and did not differ from multi-partnered heterosexuals on this score. Although lack of statistical power did not allow us to establish more clearly this result, it strongly suggests that bisexual men had not been reached by gay-oriented preventive messages to the same extent as exclusively homosexual men, this being possibly explained by their having different socio-demographic characteristics. Indeed, behavioural differences vanished when controlling for these characteristics, suggesting the important role of these latter.

**Conclusions**

Although further studies, with greater statistical power, are needed to confirm the findings tentatively described above, the data to hand do enable us to draw conclusions of public health relevance.

Since health education programmes should be carefully matched to the socio-demographic characteristics of the targeted populations (Lifson, 1992), the particular characteristics of bisexual men pose a challenge to those responsible for designing HIV prevention programmes. Bisexual men may be difficult to reach through gay community networks, not only because they do not necessarily identify themselves as gay, but also because such networks are not developed among people with many of the characteristics bisexual men in France appear to share, such as belonging to the working class or living in small provincial towns.

Such difficulties may be compounded by other factors. Recent work by Mendes-Leite (1991; Mendes-Leite and De Busscher, 1993) suggest that geographical factors may act in two rather different ways to heighten some men's HIV-related risks. First, the geographic origin of sexual partners may be used by subjects to evaluate their risk of becoming infected: men coming from outside big cities (AIDS epicentres) may be viewed as less risky, so that condom use is believed to be less necessary. Second, persons living in non-urban areas may have to travel long distances when seeking homosexual encounters. In order to balance the costliness – in all senses of the term – of their travels by having 'efficient' encounters, they may comply with safer sex guidelines less rigorously, even when they have a good knowledge of what these recommendations are. Both of these factors may be particularly relevant to bisexual men who, as our study shows, tend to live in more rural areas than exclusively homosexual men.

According to our study, bisexuals are similar to multi-partnered heterosexuals as regards the number, but not the gender, of partners and the frequency of unprotected penetrative practices; they seem to engage more frequently than exclusively homosexual men in HIV-related risk behaviours and to have less diversified preventive strategies. Other studies indicate that bisexual men, and especially those who do not identify as gay, are less likely than homosexual men to consider themselves at risk of HIV infection (Chu *et al.*, 1992; Mendes-Leite, 1992; Wood *et al.*, 1993), and are less well informed and less aware of the risks and how to avoid them (Bochow, 1990). Some of them may lead a covert homosexual life alongside an overt heterosexual life, and their female partners may be aware neither of their homosexuality, nor of their serostatus (Weatherburn *et al.*, 1990; Rogers and Turner, 1991; Chu *et al.*, 1992; Krijnen *et al.*, 1994). They themselves are likely to ignore their serostatus, as revealed in our study and in studies among gay press readers (Schiltz *et al.*, 1993). Even when they are linked to gay networks, such men are likely to adopt safer sex to a lesser extent than homosexual men, as revealed by a study of readers of a series of pamphlets targeting homosexual men (Pelé *et al.*, 1994). Some bisexual men therefore may play a role in facilitating the HIV transmission between homosexuals and heterosexuals, and in maintaining the HIV epidemic among homosexuals.

These results call for specially designed HIV prevention strategies different from those currently directed at self-identified gay men. So far in France, no preventive work targeted at bisexual men has taken place. Such work is being developed, however, and will aim to address the risks associated with unprotected anal sex in health education materials with a strong heterosexual orientation (Pelé, 1995), thus taking into account the fact that homosexual and heterosexual worlds are interwoven. The implementation of these projects is, however, dependent on government approval and funding.

## Notes

We are indebted to Françoise Magnin for typing the manuscript, and to Kim Phung Huynh for documentation facilities. The ACSF is a survey supported by the Agence Nationale de Recherches sur le Sida (ANRS), the Direction Générale de la Santé (DGS – General Health Department), the Comité Français d' Education pour la Santé (CFES) and the Agence Française de Lutte contre le Sida (AFLS).

1 The ACSF (Analyse des Comportements Sexuels en France) investigators are Alfred Spira (Director), Nathalie Bajos (Coordinator), André Béjin, Nathalie Beltzer, Michel Bozon, Béatrice Ducot, André Durandeau, Alexis Ferrand, Alain Giami, Augustin Gilloire, Michel Giraud, Henri Léridon, Dominique Ludwig, Antoine Messiah, Jean-Paul Moatti, Lise Mounnier, Hélène Olomucki, Jeanine de Poplavsky, Benoit Riandey, Brenda Spencer, Jean-Marie Sztalryd and Hubert Touzard. Collaborators are Patrick de Colomby, Jean-Marie Firdion, Françoise Le Pont and Josiane Warszawski.
2 Individuals selected by their date of birth exclusively (situation 5) served as controls relative to individuals in a potentially at-risk situation (situations 1 to 4) for the analysis for which such a dichotomy was relevant.

## References

ACSF INVESTIGATORS (1992) 'AIDS and Sexual Behaviour in France', *Nature*, 360, pp. 407–9.

BAJOS, N., BOZON, M., GIAMI, A. and FERRAND, A. (1994) 'Orientating the Research Procedure', in SPIRA, A., BAJOS, N. and the ACSF GROUP (Eds) *Sexual Behaviour and AIDS*, Aldershot, Avebury.

BOCHOW, M. (1990) 'Aids and Gay Men: Individual Strategies and Collective Coping', *European Sociological Review*, 6, pp. 181–8.

CATANIA, J. A., GIBSON, D. R., CHITWOOD, D. D. and COATES, T. J. (1990) 'Methological Problems in AIDS Behavioral Research: Influence on

Measurement Error and Participation Bias in Studies of Sexual Behavior', *Psychological Bulletin*, 108, pp. 339–62.

CHU, S. Y., PETERMAN, T. A., DOLL, L. S., BUEHLER, J. W. and CURRAN, J. W. (1992) 'AIDS in Bisexual Men in the United States: Epidemiology and Transmission to Women', *American Journal of Public Health*, 82, pp. 220–4.

COCHRAN, W. G. (1977) *Sampling Techniques*, New York, John Wiley and Sons.

EKSTRAND, M. L., COATES, T. J., GUYDISH, J. R., HAUCK, W. W., COLLETTE, L. and HULLEY, S. B. (1994) 'Are Bisexually Identified Men in San Francisco a Common Vector for Spreading HIV Infection to Women?', *American Journal of Public Health*, 84, pp. 915–19.

KRIJNEN, P., VAN DEN HOEK, J. A. R. and COUTINHO, R. A. (1994) 'Do Bisexual Men Play a Significant Role in the Heterosexual Spread of HIV?', *Sexually Transmitted Diseases*, 21, pp. 24–5.

LAGRANGE, H. (1991) 'Le nombre de partenaires sexuels: les hommes en ont-ils plus que les femmes?', *Population*, 2, pp. 249–78.

LEE, E. S., FORTHOFER, R. N. and LORIMER, R. J. (1989) *Analysing Complex Survey Data*, London, Sage.

LÉRIDON, H. (1989) 'Comportements sexuels et Sida en France', *Contraception Fertilité Sexualité*, 17, pp. 919–24.

LÉRIDON, H. and BOZON, M. (1993) 'Présentation de l'enquête ACSF', *Population*, 48, 1197–204.

LHOMOND, B. (1993) 'Les enquêtes sur les comportements sexuels de Kinsey au rapport gai', *Sociétés*, 39, pp. 29–38.

LIFSON, A. R. (1992) 'Men who Have Sex with Men: Continued Challenges for Preventing HIV Infection and AIDS', *American Journal of Public Health*, 82, pp. 166–7.

MENDES-LEITE, R. (1991) 'La culture des sexualités à l'époque du Sida: représentations, comportements et pratiques (homo) sexuelles', *Homosexualités et Sida*, Lille, Cahiers Gai-Kitsch-Camp, Université 4, pp. 151–64.

MENDES-LEITE, R. (1992) 'Pratiques à risque: les fictions dangereuses', *Le Journal du Sida*, 42, pp. 44–5.

MENDES-LEITE, R. and DE BUSSCHER, P. O. (1993) 'Homosexuels et VIH: influence des facteurs géographiques sur la prise de risque', *Transcriptase*, 12, pp. 10–13.

MESSIAH, A. and MOURET-FOURME, E. (1993) 'Homosexualité, bisexualité: éléments de socio-biographie sexuelle', *Population*, 48, pp. 1353–80.

MESSIAH, A., MOURET-FOURME, E., PELLETIER, A. and the ACSF GROUP (1994) 'Socio-Demographic Characteristics and Sexual Behaviour of Bisexual Men, Compared with Homosexual and Heterosexual Men: Results from the French National Survey on Sexual Behaviour', paper presented at AIDS in Europe: The Behavioural Aspect, European Conference on Methods and Results of Psycho-Social AIDS Research, Berlin, 26–29 September.

MESSIAH, A., MOURET-FOURME, E. and the ACSF GROUP (1995) 'Socio-Demographic Characteristics and Sexual Behaviour of Bisexual Men: Implications for HIV/STD Transmission and Prevention', *American Journal of Public Health,* 85, pp. 1543–46.

MESSIAH, A., PELLETIER, A. and the ACSF GROUP (1996) 'Partner-Specific Sexual Practices among Heterosexual Women and Men with Multiple Partners: Results from the French National Survey', ACSF, *Archives of Sexual Behaviour,* 25, pp. 233–47.

PELÉ, G. (1995) Personal communication. Direction Générale de la Santé, Ministère des Affaires Sociales et de la Santé, France.

PELÉ, G., ANGUENOT, M., CHARFE, Y. *et al.* (1994) 'Pamphlets Targetting Homosexual Men in France: Acceptance and Impact on Risk Behaviors', Xth International Conference on AIDS, Yokohama, Japan, 7–12 August. Abstract 172D.

POLLAK, M. (1982) 'L'homosexualité masculine, ou: le bonheur dans le ghetto?', *Sexualités Occidentales,* Communications, 35 Paris, Point Seuil, pp. 56–80.

POLLAK, M. (1988) *Les homosexuels et le SIDA: sociologie d'une épidémie,* Paris, A. M. Métailié.

POLLAK, M. (1991) 'La diffusion hétérogène du safer sex', *Le Journal du Sida,* 31–32, Suppl., pp. 27–9.

POLLAK, M. and SCHILTZ, M. A. (1987) 'Identité sociale et gestion d'un risque de santé. Les homosexuels face au SIDA', *Actes de la Recherche en Sciences Sociales,* 68, pp. 77–102.

POLLAK, M. and SCHILTZ, M. A. (1991a) 'Six années d'enquête sur les homo- et bisexuels masculins face au Sida: livre des données', *Bulletin de Methodologie Sociologique,* 31, pp. 32–48.

POLLAK, M. and SCHILTZ, M. A. (1991b) 'Six années d'enquête sur les homo- et bisexuels masculins face au Sida', Rapport à l'Agence Nationale de Recherche sur le Sida (ANRS), Paris, ANRS.

POLLAK, M. and SCHILTZ, M. A. (1991c) 'Les homosexuels français face au Sida: modifications des pratiques sexuelles et émergence de nouvelles valeurs', *Anthropologie et Sociétés,* 15, pp. 53–65.

RÉSEAU NATIONAL DE SANTÉ PUBLIQUE (1994) 'Surveillance du Sida en France: situation au 30 septembre 1994', *Bulletin Épidémiologique Hebdomadair,* 45, pp. 209–15.

ROGERS, S. M. and TURNER, C. F. (1991) 'Male-Male Sexual Contact in the U.S.A.: Findings from Five Sample Surveys, 1970–1990', *Journal of Sex Research,* 28, pp. 491–519.

SCHILTZ, M. A. (1993) *Les homosexuels masculins face au Sida: enquêtes 1991–1992,* Rapport de fin de contrat à l'Agence Nationale de Recherche sur le Sida, Paris.

SCHILTZ, M. A., CHARFE, Y. and DORÉ, V. (1993) *Les premiers résultats de l'enquête 1993 auprès des lecteurs de la presse homosexuelle,* Rapport à l'Agence Nationale de Recherche sur le Sida (ANRS), November, Paris, ANRS.

SCHMIDT, W. K., KRASNIK, A., BRENDSTRUP, E., ZOFFMANN, H. and LARSEN, S. O. (1989) 'Occurrence of Sexual Behaviour Related to the Risk of HIV-Infection: A Survey Among Danish Men, 16–55 Years of Age', *Danish Medical Bulletin*, 36, pp. 84–8.

SHAH, B. V., BARNWELL, B. G., NILEEN HUNT, P. and LaVANGE, L. M. (1993) *Sudaan: Professional Software for Survey Data Analysis for Multi-Stage Sample Designs*, Release 6.34 (September 1993), Research Triangle Park, Research Triangle Institute.

SIMON, P., GONDONNEAU, J., MIRONER, L. and DOURLEN-ROLLIER, A. M. (1972), 'L'homosexualité', *Rapport sur le comportement sexuel des français*, Paris, René Juillard et Pierre Charron, pp. 266–71.

SMITH, T. W. (1991) 'Adult Sexual Behavior in 1989: Number of Partners, Frequency of Intercourse and Risk of AIDS', *Family Planning Perspectives*, 23, pp. 102–7.

SPIRA, A., BAJOS, N. and the ACSF GROUP (Eds) (1994) *Sexual Behaviour and AIDS*, Aldershot, Avebury.

UPCHURCH, D. M., WEISMAN, C. S., SHEPHERD, M. *et al.* (1991) 'Interpartner Reliability of Reporting of Recent Sexual Behaviors', *American Journal of Epidemiology*, 134, pp. 1159–66.

WEATHERBURN, P., DAVIES, P. M., HUNT, A. J., COXON, A. P. M. and McMANUS, T. J. (1990) 'Heterosexual Behaviour in a Large Cohort of Homosexually Active Men in England and Wales', *AIDS Care*, 2, pp. 319–24.

WELLINGS, K., WADSWORTH, J. and JOHNSON, A. (1994) *Sexual Attitudes and Lifestyles*, Oxford, Blackwell Scientific Publications.

WOOD, R. W., KRUEGER, L. E., PEARLMAN, T. C. and GOLDBAUM, G. (1993) 'HIV Transmission: Women's Risk from Bisexual Men', *American Journal of Public Health*, 83, pp. 1757–9.

# Chapter 5

## Bisexuality and HIV/AIDS in Mexico

*Ana Luisa Liguori*
*with Miguel González Block and Peter Aggleton*[1]

*Cuál es la diferencia entre un mexicano homosexual y uno que no lo es? Dos copas.* (Chiste popular)[2]

A few years prior to the research into male sexual culture in Mexico that is described in this chapter, an architect had mentioned to Miguel González Block that it could be important to carry out a study on sexually transmitted diseases (STDs) among construction workers since, in his many years of professional experience, he had noticed that building workers sometimes had sexual relationships with each other. Before the widespread emergence of AIDS in Mexico, we decided that it would be worthwhile conducting research on this topic, particularly since some of the key features of sexual culture among construction workers might be relatively widespread among men from the lower social strata more generally.

An initial review of officially registered cases of AIDS suggested that while at the time there was a higher reported prevalence of disease among the higher social strata, the epidemic was growing more rapidly among the lower socio-economic groups. Additionally, while the proportion of cases of AIDS ascribed to homosexual activity was higher in the middle and higher strata than in the lower strata, the likely risk of transmission through bisexual activity was greater in the lower strata than in the middle or higher strata. These findings reinforced our decision to carry out exploratory research among construction workers. We were particularly interested in studying men who had sex with other men but who identified themselves as being heterosexual.

In daily life, frequent reference is made to such behaviour. In Mexico, sexual play of a verbal and even physical nature is very evident among groups of men in *pulquerías*[3] or in workplaces where there is a predominantly male presence. It is accompanied by a kind of comradeship and complicity where, in addition to talk about sexual exploits (both alleged and real), there is an atmosphere charged with sexuality. At the level of popular culture, there is much talk of *machos calados* or *machos probados* – men who are very macho, so macho in fact that they have sexual relations with men as well as with women. Such men are always assumed to take the active role, this action in no way detracting from their masculinity. Academically, however, little has been written about such behaviour. Indeed, an initial bibliographical search on Mexican sexual culture was both unproductive and frustrating. There was virtually nothing at all on the subject. What could be found came from three main sources – literature, a few published research studies, and preliminary enquiries linked to the government's National AIDS Control Programme (CONASIDA). Before describing our own research, we will examine what can be learned from each of these sources.

### Literary Responses

*¿quién es totalmente buga? nadie ¿verdad?*[4] (Luis Zapata, *El vampiro de la colonia Roma*)

In his essay *El laberinto de la soledad*, Octavio Paz (1950) analyses the historical origins of Mexican culture and, in some chapters of the book, ideal attributes for men and for women. For a Mexican man, his manliness is paramount, something he never gives up. He is stoic, inscrutable and looks upon death with contempt. He is also a liar, but lies not only to deceive others, but above all, to deceive himself. In Mexican culture, everything associated with masculinity is praised, in the same way as everything associated with femininity is scorned. Because of this, the masculine homosexual is regarded with a certain indulgence, because he is the active party. Conversely, the passive one is viewed as a degraded and despicable being.

This ambiguity of thought, according to Paz, is evident in the wordplay or verbal combat that takes place between men, involving an exchange of obscene references and double meanings in which the loser, the one who in the end cannot answer back, is possessed or violated by the other, as spectators look on and laugh. In his reflections on the essentially Mexican word *chingar*, Paz explores its many and varied meanings. Defined in the dictionary as a vulgar expression 'to fuck', *chingar* is to exercise violence over another person. An active masculine verb with connotations of cruelty, stinging, ripping apart and staining, the idea of violation runs throughout all its meanings. Paz is of the opinion that the Mexican man has certain homosexual inclinations which show themselves in, among other things, his liking for exclusively male groups. But whatever the origin of these attitudes, the essential attribute of the macho man, strength, is nearly always manifested in the capacity to wound or tear apart, wipe out, or humiliate – in other words, in his ability to 'fuck' the other person.

There also exist other literary texts that illustrate the theme of bisexuality in Mexico. In 1964 Vincente Leñero published his novel *Los albañiles*. In it an elderly watchman or security guard is murdered on a building site. Most of the book describes the characters on the building site who could have had a motive for killing him. The old man, don Jesús, is a person who deliberately gives the impression of being ill and helpless, but in fact always tries to do harm to those around him. The person over whom he has most influence is Isidro, a 15-year-old labourer, who he entertains and involves in his stories.

The young man stays many nights to share a drink with him. Throughout most of the novel it is clear that the older man has sexual relations with Isidro, while at the same time he is advising him how to treat women and how to make himself irresistible to his girlfriend. Taking advantage of the trust the young man has in him, he asks him to bring his girlfriend round and leave them alone for a while so he can advise her too. The old man takes the opportunity to rape the girl. When Isidro challenges don Jesús' actions, the old man humiliates him saying, 'I forgot to tell you one thing, what we call people like you is queers' (Leñero, 1964, p. 158). When the murder investigation is carried out and Isidro is suspected, the detective says to him, 'the watchman had to explain to you what women are like, he had to teach you the caresses that you should use to make them loose, he did the same with you himself'. Then he accuses him of having killed don Jesús to show the other building workers that, above all, he is not queer.

Luis Zapata's novel *El vampiro de la colonia Roma* contains several notable references to bisexuality. At one point the main character in the novel, Adonis, turns to prostitution. One of his many clients tells him that he is currently going out with a man and with a woman. The man wants the relationship to become more steady or stable, but he is resisting, because as he says 'I have my girlfriend, and I don't want to betray her' (Zapata, 1979, p. 82). Towards the end of the novel, this same character talks about a new neighbourhood he has moved to. He says 'it is the most homosexual in Mexico, there are hundreds of gay guys on every block, and that is without counting those who are not gay but who will screw with you anyway'.

A third illustration of behavioural bisexuality can be found in the story *El Rayo Macoy* by Rafael Ramírez Heredia. Published in 1984, this describes how a man of humble origins rises to become a successful boxer and national champion (Ramírez, 1984). One night he goes out to a nightclub with a gang of close friends. While there, he notices a blonde woman. One of his friends warns him to be careful because the blonde is a man. Rayo, the character, simply shrugs his shoulders and rubs his crotch. Between bursts of laughter he says, so long as the hole is white-skinned it does not matter whose it is. Towards the end of the story, on a trip to Acapulco, on impulse he marries a cabaret star. Instead of making love to her for the first time, he leaves to go out partying with his male friends. The story finishes at this party with Rayo kissing Cascabel the transvestite on the mouth, sharing the same drink with him and undressing him.

### The View from Research

*Cualquier hoyo, aunque sea de pollo* (refran popular)[5]

Turning now to the more academic literature, when we first began our enquiries, there were few relevant references on sexuality in general, or to male bisexuality in particular. Perhaps the only exception were studies carried out by Carrier (1985, 1989a, 1989b), Lumsden (1991) and Prieur (1994a), although as our study got under way, a small number of other investigations came to be funded as part of the government's National AIDS Control Programme (CONASIDA).

Carrier began his work in Mexico in 1968, long before the first cases of AIDS were recorded. Along with Lumsden and Prieur, he was interested in the social construction of various 'sexual types'. All shared the view that the cultural ideals which regulate sexual roles and behaviour in Mexican society are rigid and stereotyped, resulting in a dual male standard related to sex, and determining the various identities available to men who have sex with other men. Carrier conducted his fieldwork in Guadalajara, Lumsden in Mexico City, and Prieur in Netzahualcóyotl, an urban area adjacent to Mexico City. All employed qualitative research techniques, in particular participant observation.

In their analyses, all three authors point to the exaggerated value given, not just to masculinity, but to hyper-masculinity in Mexico. As a result, everything feminine or female is devalued, including effeminate men and homosexuals. In Mexico, it is very easy for men to have sexual relations with other men. What makes this behaviour possible is the fact that the man who participates in these relationships is not stigmatized so long as he performs an active role. His behaviour is not considered homosexual, nor is his masculine self-image threatened. Indeed, having sex in this way with other men may in fact reaffirm his masculinity as the penetrator of others. The opposite is true from the man who allows himself to be penetrated. He is the only one likely to be seen a homosexual.

The existence of these social roles and identities means that high value is placed on anal sex in sexual relations between men, with men tending to specialize in roles, either as the penetrator or the penetrated. If one individual plays both parts, he tends not to do so with the same person. Often, what determines who penetrates, and who allows himself to be penetrated, is which man is the most feminine. This idea is confirmed by the fact that those men who perform both roles are said to be *internacionales* – a term which, according to Carrier, emphasizes the supposedly 'foreign' origins of this practice (Carrier, 1989b). Whether, as is claimed, up to 30 per cent of Mexican men between 15 and 25 years of age have some history of bisexual relationships (Carrier, 1985), is open to debate. Nevertheless, the existence of such patterns of behaviour, in the absence of clearly defined homosexual or bisexual *identities*, has important implications for HIV prevention, as we will see later.

Unlike either Carrier or Prieur, Lumsden attempts to trace the origins of contemporary patterns of sexual culture to the impact of colonialism on pre-Hispanic culture. He argues that it was during colonialism that the very stereotyped and rigid roles that now exist in Mexico began to be constructed. For Lumsden, the macho stance of the male is associated with the mentality of the conqueror through its emphasis on invulnerability and the obligation to abuse the weakest. The macho man having sexual relations in an active role with a 'passive' homosexual is therefore merely taking advantage of an opportunity which has been presented to him, and doing so does not call into question his masculinity (Lumsden, 1991).

In more recent time, social class, degree of remoteness from place of origin and the North American gay movement have all influenced homosexual and bisexual practice in Mexico. As a result, the identities of men who have sex with other men vary greatly. Lumsden classifies them as country or rural/indigenous, urban/provincial, and metropolitan/cosmopolitan. In general, a complex set of values condition the expressions of homosexuality both publicly and privately that now predominate.

> Bisexuality takes a variety of forms in Mexico, ranging from married males who have homosexual partners on the side, and are conscious that they eroticise other males, to the *mayates*[6] who only have sex in return for some material inducement, and the *bugas*[7] who only do so after having got drunk. In between there are considerable numbers who frequently have sex with other males without ever questioning their sexuality in the process. (Lumsden, 1991, p. 46)

The research of the Norwegian sociologist Prieur was carried out between 1988 and 1992. Her object of study was a group of homosexual men from extremely low socio-economic backgrounds, most of whom were transvestite or of very feminine or effeminate appearance, and many of whom were male prostitutes. Prieur conducted an ethnographic study of this group looking at a wide range of issues including the relationship between men who had sexual relationships with the 'girls' in this group but who considered themselves to be, and were socially seen as, heterosexual (or *mayates*). For Prieur, the exaggerated femininity of the men she studied was a response to the rigid construction of sexual roles; such 'femininity' was being used to attract men, and to signal sexual availability. Often transvestites show off their ability to get off with 'true men'. The more masculine their partner, the more feminine they feel. Such homosexuals often live for long periods of time with men who then leave them to get married or have sex with a woman. In such relationships, transvestites generally take the passive role, or at least pretend to do so.

While men can have sexual relations with an effeminate man without being considered homosexual, and without having overt conflicts of identity, to say that such behaviour is not stigmatized is an oversimplification. Contact between 'heterosexual' men and homosexual men can only occur in specialized contexts (such as bars) where the transvestites go. It is not that the feminine appearance of the homosexual men deceives the supposedly 'heterosexual' partner, it is more likely that the latter is deceiving himself. For Prieur, it is no coincidence that much of the communication surrounding such relationships is non-verbal, implying a semi-consciousness on the part of transvestites' partners. We may be dealing here with a group of men who justify their sexual behaviour by the fact that so many of them do it, rather than because it is morally acceptable. Although they rarely admit to it, many transvestite informants stated that there are *mayates* who allow themselves to be penetrated. The processes of individual and social denial that operate in and around such relationships pose particular challenges for HIV prevention.

Further insight into the processes at work in such denial comes from recent work by Hernández (1994) in the state of Veracruz. Through individual and focus group interviews from young men, data are being collected on the ways in which the stigma of homosexuality, and the dread of being perceived as homosexual, may structure the development of masculinity. Because of the strength with which homosexuality is stigmatized, young men may use a range of strategies to deny their same-sex desires and practices, and to demonstrate their manhood. These can vary from efforts to conceal their homosexual behaviour from public view, to not carrying condoms when going to have sex with another man (as this might imply a level of acceptance or pre-planning or awareness of such behaviour), to making a woman pregnant. The focus of this research is on the ways in which stigma about homosexuality may heighten sexual health risks, particularly among behaviourally bisexual men who consider themselves to be heterosexual.

### A Government View

Within the framework of government efforts to reduce the impact of the AIDS epidemic in Mexico, further research into male bisexuality has been carried out. Much of this research has been carried out with the support of CONASIDA. Both the National Institute of Public Health (INSP) and the National Institute of Epidemiological Diagnosis and Registration (INDRE), for example, have given much time to identifying patterns of sexual behaviour so as to project the growth of the epidemic and facilitate the development of educational programmes for prevention.

In contrast to the more qualitative kinds of enquiry described above which tend to have focused on the meanings linked to bisexual practice and the cultures within which it occurs, the majority of these studies have aimed to measure the incidence and correlates of bisexual behaviours through studies of Knowledge, Attitudes, Beliefs and reported Practices (KABP). From 1988 onwards, a number of such studies were conducted among behaviourally homosexual and bisexual men, most frequently recruited through gay community groups and through centres where men go to be tested for HIV. Table 5.1 lists some of these investigations.

Summary articles based on this and other work have been produced by García *et al.* (1991), who offer a preliminary typology of forms of bisexuality in Mexico, and discuss the possible implications of the forms they detect for HIV prevention work, and by Izazola (1994). Subsequent enquiry by Izazola and Tolbert (in CONASIDA, 1994) has involved focus group discussions with

*Table 5.1 KABP Studies in Mexico*

| Article | Type of research | n | Place of recruitment | % reporting bisexual behaviour | % HIV positive | % reported use of condom |
|---|---|---|---|---|---|---|
| Secretaria de Salud, 1988 | KABP study on self-identified homosexual/ bisexual men. Lacks represent-ativeness. | 852 in 1987, 715 in 1988, total 1568 | 6 Mexican cities, places frequented by homosexual men, bars, etc. | 51% | 75% agreed to take test, 19% positive in 1987, 11% positive in 1988. | Sometimes 59%, in last 4 months 44%, in last month 34%. |
| Izazola *et al*, 1988 | Self-identified homosexual and bisexual men. Lacks represent-ativeness | 340 | Mexico DF, through gay community and places frequented by homosexuals. | 56% | 1985 15%, 1986 23%, 1987 39.1% | Not reported. |
| Izazola *et al*, 1991 | Self-identified bisexual men. Lacks represent-ativeness. | | 6 Mexican cities. Places frequented by homosexuals. | 27% | 2–25%, depending on city. Exclusively insertive or exclusively receptive behaviour associated with lower incidence than mixed behaviour. | 30% |
| Hernández *et al*, 1992 | HIV incidence and sexual behaviour survey. | 2,314 | CONASIDA information and detection centre. | 24% | 21% of bisexuals, 34% of homosexuals. Among those with | 5% among those who were receptive only. |

| | | | | | | |
|---|---|---|---|---|---|---|
| | Self-selected sample. | | | | exclusively receptive or exclusively insertive behaviour, lower incidence of HIV than among those with mixed behaviour. | |
| Ramírez *et al.*, 1994 | Knowledge of AIDS. Interviews on sexual conduct. Correlates insertive and receptive behaviour with homosexual and bisexual identity. Self-identified sample. | 200 | Bars, restaurants and homes of people who agreed to be interviewed. | 29% | Not measured. | Insertive anal sex: 45% used often; 30% occasional use; 25% never. Receptive anal sex: 46% frequently; 27% occasional use; 27% never. |
| CONASIDA, 1994 | Representative sample of men 15–60 years of age, Mexico DF and urban area. | 13,197 | Homes. | Four categories of bisexual behaviour, 2.1% in last year. | Not measured. | Of those who had sex with both sexes in last year, 13.9% used condom with men and women in last sexual relationship, and 4% used one with men but not with women. |

behaviourally bisexual men and has led to the development of educational videos for HIV prevention that deal with the subject of bisexuality (e.g. *De chile, de dulce y de manteca*).[8]

## Agreements, Differences and Questions

There are elements of continuity and discontinuity in the studies and reports cited above. It is clear that in Mexico today a not insignificant number of men who consider themselves to be heterosexual have sex with other men, and that a relatively high percentage of men who identify themselves as homosexual have had, or have, sexual relations with women. What is less clear is the relative importance of this bisexual behaviour for HIV transmission (Garcia *et al.*, 1991; Hernández *et al.*, 1992, p. 58), especially since there is evidence to suggest that bisexually active men may have a slightly lower probability of infection than men with exclusively homosexual behaviour (Hernández, 1992, p. 893). We also know little about the relative risks confronting men who are both insertive and receptive in their sexual relations with other men compared to those who do not display this versatility of role (Izazola *et al.*, 1991; Hernández *et al.*, 1992).

## 'Bisexuality' among Construction Workers in Mexico

*Con un abañil que esté bueno todas decimos: ay pues ya bañadito yo me lo echo, y a últimas ya ni bañadito. Ya con el vino hasta se olvidó el baño.*[9]
(Vanessa, a transvestite)

In contrast to the studies so far described, the work we conducted among construction workers does not look at self-identified groups who practise homosexual behaviour, nor those who consider themselves to be at special risk (González Block and Liguori, 1992). Instead it tackles questions of bisexuality in Mexico by looking at a group of men who identify themselves as heterosexual and who without doubt share characteristics with many other men from similar backgrounds. Such men may have an active sexuality, but face restrictions on their access to potential heterosexual partners (through economic limitation or through temporary migration), while living in often overcrowded conditions, and within a culture that does not especially stigmatize sex between men so long as the individual concerned acts as the penetrator of another.

### Methodology

In order to better understand sexual culture within the daily lives of building workers, participant observation and key informant interviews were identified as the most appropriate data collection methods. In order to select an appropriate construction project, advice was first sought from experts within the construction industry. Construction projects vary from the smallest, carried out without an architect and with just a few building workers, to vast buildings employing a team of architects and engineers and up to 3,000 or more building workers. On medium-sized sites with fewer than a hundred building workers, there may be a number of foremen. On smaller sites, there is just one foreman who supervises the workers. In very large projects, the work is organized by façades, by floors or by sections, with each group or façade having a supervisor or overseer.

The advisers recommended selecting a project with no more than a hundred building workers, which would facilitate observation and avoid unnecessary hazards to the investigator. On large projects, accidents are frequent, including deliberate ones. Even architects refrain from visiting such projects alone after working hours, because the site is transformed into a world alien to them: it is the home of building workers and labourers, who come seasonally from the provinces and have no money. After six in the evening – especially on Saturdays, which are paydays – it is common for many of them to play cards and drink. Occasionally they invite women or homosexual men. There are frequent fights. The larger the building site, the more complex its social network. A construction project for a horizontal condominium of ten houses was selected, which we will call 'San Carlos', in the Magdalena Contreras District. During the study, the number of building workers fluctuated between fifty and a hundred, depending on the capital flow.

Participant observation requires prolonged contact with those observed, in a role they recognize. It was carried out in this study by a young male social scientist working with us who had received special training in how to assume an acceptable role among the workers. For the purposes of this chapter, we will call him Francisco.

The project was presented initially to the site foreman in order to gain his support. The site foreman appointed Francisco as assistant to his son-in-law, who supervised the staff and kept control over output. Francisco went to work regularly, working the normal hours from eight in the morning until six in the evening. Although the building workers noticed that Francisco was not a labourer, his personality and his daily presence enabled him to gain acceptance.

Fieldwork was carried out between November 1989 and February 1990 and focused on twenty-two workers of different ages, with different incomes and trades, and from different places of origin. Data were collected on, among other things, migratory history, characteristics of their dwelling, expenditure and social interaction, with particular attention being given to physical and verbal manifestations of sexuality. Of the twenty-two building workers studied, four were key informants and provided the majority of the information on sexual values and conduct, and on the role of bisexuality in their lives. Francisco accompanied the building workers to a *pulque* bar at mealtimes, and sometimes stayed on the site after work to socialize with the men. He also sought opportunities to go out with some of them at weekends.

## Work Organization

Generally speaking, the architects do not recruit the workers or deal directly with them. This is delegated to a site foreman or contractor who is responsible for supervising the staff. Site foremen are very powerful, since they mediate between the architects and workers, organize the work, have the power to dismiss workers who present a problem and, above all, pay the wages. The contractor never works on the site: this would demean him and diminish his power over his subordinates; but he must *know* everything related to the building trade, so that if any of his workers does something wrong, he can correct him and oblige him to put it right. For example, if he sees that they are building a wall wrongly, he knocks it over, lays a few bricks to show how it is done and immediately goes away. The contractor usually has an overseer, who is the person in whom he puts his trust; the latter represents him on the site and is responsible for watching over things and solving problems when the contractor is not there.

The project selected for the research was in the hands of the group of architects who had designed it and they were supervising its progress daily. They were assisted by a 'resident', a young architect who had recently graduated and who stayed on the site all day. The residents need to have the right character to run a site. At San Carlos, the first resident contracted gave up because he could not stand the work dynamics. Afterwards, the foremen joked about him saying, 'We killed that architect' and 'That one couldn't stand the pace because we *screwed* him'.

Below the resident were two foremen contractors, who carried out the functions described above. At the next level were the skilled workers: bricklayers, carpenters, plasterers, tilers, etc. Plumbers, electricians and blacksmiths do not generally form part of the big 'clans' of building workers, because these jobs are subcontracted. Among the skilled workers, the best paid are those who do the finishing, since it is their work that the client sees. The architects refer to them as the 'stars' of the site. At the bottom of the hierarchy are the labourers, who are the worst paid and carry out the hardest and most dangerous work. Most of the skilled workers start as labourers. The cleverest of them learn the skill quickly, and some of them manage to purchase their working tools (although these are expensive) and rise in the labour hierarchy.

At the start of the week, the foreman organizes working teams made up of a skilled worker and a labourer, in order to achieve the best output. Sometimes a labourer works with the same skilled worker for several weeks, but as a rule the foreman changes the teams frequently so that excessive familiarity will not slow down the work. The skilled worker puts a lot of pressure on the labourer, because he (the skilled worker) is generally paid at piece-work rates. If the labourer does not work efficiently, the skilled worker asks for another assistant. The labourer, on the other hand, cannot request a move to another team. His basic task consists of bringing the skilled worker all the materials he needs to do his work. The labourer must work quickly, so that the skilled worker achieves the maximum output. The labourer is also responsible for sweeping, cleaning and removing rubbish. A bricklayer never does a labourer's work, because that would diminish his status. Generally speaking, the labourer does not do the work of the skilled worker either. If the skilled worker has confidence in the labourer and is absent for some reason, the labourer may dare to experiment with the trowel and lay a few bricks. On his return, the skilled worker usually boasts of having taught him the job, but then says he has done it badly. Besides doing their work, the labourers have to provide the skilled worker with personal services, such as buying food or running errands.

Between the skilled worker and the labourer there is frequently an ambivalent relationship. On the one hand, it is one of protection, on the other hand, one of subjection. Paternalism and authoritarianism go hand in hand. Generally speaking, the skilled workers try to make life difficult for the labourers of other skilled workers. Each one defends his own labourer, but he does this because the labourer is the only person he can give orders to on the site, so he cannot afford to lose his authority over him. And while each skilled worker defends his labourer against the others, he is generally demanding and hard on his subordinate, and may even maltreat him. The following example provides an illustration of this type of relationship.

Gonzalo[10] is a bricklayer who is building a wall; his labourer is bringing him the water he needs.

'Hey you, bring me some more water, that old bugger [referring to a labourer who had been helping him and whom he had asked to have replaced] is a real lazy sod.'

'Where did you send him?'

'I threw the bastard out, we're divorced.'

'Didn't you like him?'

'Not likely. I divorced him, to hell with him.'

'Is it here that you want the water?'

The labourer brings the water and goes to fetch some stones.

'I chucked that old bastard out, granddad, he doesn't give me a hard-on any more, he doesn't do a stroke for me.'

'Can't you get it up any more?'

'Not with him I can't. He's a drunken old sod just like you.'

'What's up boss? Since when do we get along this way?'

'Next thing, you'll be telling me you don't drink.'

'Well, I like my drop of *pulque*, but I don't get as pissed as him.'

'But you're even getting too big for your boots already! Hand me that stone before you make me get mad; that one's fine, I just stick it in there, see.'

Gonzalo then starts talking to another skilled worker called Nicolás, who is nearby laying bricks.

'Isn't it true that I chucked out the old man because he is a queer!'

'For being a queer and a bad friend. He's no good for anything. Now they've sent me another one, but I think he's as bad as the other drunken bastard.'

'Like a woman when she's untamed, you have to break the bugger in.'

'Look at the ham-fisted way he's loading those bloody pebbles,' he says, pointing to his labourer who is loading some rocks.

The labourer, who is really straining himself, replies, 'Pebbles? I'd like to see you load them.'

'That's what you're my labourer for, so that you can bring me some bloody great rocks. Here bend down and hold this [referring to a piece of wire he is positioning] for me; not so tight, if you squeeze it I won't have enough for you. There, pull on it, that's enough.'

The labourer turns to him. 'Do you want more water?'

'No, you'd better go and get me a soft drink.'

'And one for me?'

'Do you think I'm paying for your keep? If there's enough money left, buy yourself one.'

### Sexuality and Daily Life on the Building Site

Work on a building site is carried out amidst insults, sexual games and '*albures*' (plays on words with a sexual content). Generally a verbal challenge develops between two men, with the aim of establishing who *penetrates* whom. It is a game demanding subtlety and quick-wittedness. The one who is left unable to reply loses and is metaphorically penetrated by the other. Frequently, they pass around phallic objects, for example, they pick up pieces of wood or make penises out of plaster and pass them to an absent-minded workmate saying: 'Look, here's a little present for you', or 'This is for you', or 'Hold this for me', etc. The other will try to avoid taking it. While chatting on the site, constant references are made to 18.5 centimetres. Whenever a reference is made to this measurement in a conversation, it produces smiles and jokes. The workers on the site regard 18.5 cm as the ideal length for a penis.

The hierarchy on the site extends to the realm of the double meaning, and this strengthens the pyramidal organization. Those in a higher position have absolute freedom to make plays on words to their subordinates. The latter, on the other hand, do not have the same opportunities to reply.

Generally speaking, the foremen take little part in this game; the double meaning finds its best expression among the skilled workers, above all when they address the labourers. The labourers cannot easily answer back. The skilled worker says things to the labourer with a double meaning, such as 'hand them to me', 'loosen this rope for me', 'get it out for me', 'now you can come', 'grab hold of it for me', 'don't move or you'll bend it', etc. Those who are best at *albures* gain the admiration of their workmates and even win the respect of the foreman because, in the event of an argument, they can undermine other workers' loyalty to him.

There are constant sexual games among the workers on the site. For example, when one worker sees another bending down, he rubs up against him or pokes him in the buttocks, either with his fingers or with some phallic object. It is also common for them to touch each other's buttocks, a practice described as *tortear*, or kneading. When asked what *tortear* meant, workers replied 'stroking the buttocks', 'grabbing the arse', 'fuck you', 'grabbing pussy'. The rules for *tortear* are similar to those for double meanings: it is done to someone of the same or lower status. The contractor does not take part in this practice. The responses of the victim vary. Some move away and try to ignore it, but others may turn round, thrust their hips forward and say 'Now grab that' or 'Come on then you bastard'.

Men working on the site constantly brag about their sexual adventures, both past and present; about the rapes they have committed, visits to prostitutes and sometimes the existence of more than one family. As regards visits to brothels or relations with prostitutes, most of them do not go because of lack of money. Others say they keep away from prostitutes for fear of AIDS. Ignacio, for example, a 45-year-old blacksmith who married at the age of 18, has always gone to prostitutes. He has worked in many parts of the country and says 'I've always had loads of opportunities.' He recounted how when he was working at a sawmill in Michoacán, his employers had a truck and sometimes took him to the red light districts. Afterwards, when he was living in Morelia, he went to the red light district there once a week. Now he just goes occasionally to the Estado de México, because he does not like the prostitutes in Mexico City.

Candelario, a 57-year-old bricklayer, said he was a great womanizer when he was young:

> I was as horny as you can get, used to have four women at the same
> time, I was a real stud. Now all that's finished, although I still make
> it with anything that's going.

However, he has calmed down now because he has two wives. He has eight children by the one he lives with and two by the other. He visits the latter twice a week, and has set them both up in homes. He says:

> I used to like going out with women, dancing and screwing; but now
> I've got two old women, it's all over.

89

The sexual adventures workers recount include those with other men. Nicolás, a master bricklayer, and married, told how:

> Not long ago, some bugger took a couple of birds on at the site. Another bugger starts touching them up and says 'Shit, they're queers. Well, what the heck.' So we stuck it up them. They wanted to screw, so why waste time?

The same informant reported that many years ago, he had 'screwed a boy':

> When I was about 24, I got pissed one day and went round to see this widow who had a son of about 14. I'd meant to fuck her, but as she wasn't there I screwed the boy instead. Now they tell me he's married but he still likes a bit of cock.

Nicolás said he had had many adventures in his life and had 'loads of skirt'. He related that on one occasion he picked up two young girls and had sex with both of them: 'One of them was pregnant . . . but what can you do? . . . Tarts are so tasty'.

Juan Daniel is a driver who delivers materials to the site. He is 27 years old and says:

> Us truck-drivers get loads of women. We take anything, old ones, skinny ones, nice ones, pretty ones, ugly ones, anything. And if a queer fancies it, I'll even screw one of them.

He goes on: 'In Veracruz, there are loads of queers, but there I only screwed one.' When asked if he liked them penetrating him, he replied 'I like screwing them, but for them to give it to me, not bloody likely!'

Timoteo is a carpenter from Poza Rica, who comes to work in Mexico City and is married. He told of his adventures one rainy day when the workmen had to stop working for a while and lit a fire. He says he used to visit the red light districts a lot, but he also had sexual relations with men: 'In Tabasco, I was with some queers who even moaned, the mother fuckers'. Ten years ago he had sexual relations with a priest:

> One day in Poza Rica, the priest was officiating at midnight mass. I was with him, because I was an altar boy. When the mass was over, I fell asleep. It was about two in the morning. It must have been about three when the priest showed up and started fondling me, and I pretended I wasn't interested, but in the end I stuck it up him.

All the listeners laughed, and he concluded: 'Poor old bugger of a priest.' He went on to say that about six months before this he had had another experience:

I was on my way home to sleep at about ten at night. There was a fair-haired boy of about 14 going the same way. I invited him to my place. There, I started fondling him, but he was scared. He told me he had never done it, but I carried on until I screwed him. Lately, no one has wanted it, but if anyone does I give it to him.

José, who is a plumber and comes from Oaxaca, says:

At the age of 12, I got my first hole. At 18 I was screwing every weekend: anything, anywhere. At work, loads of tarts: women working as painters, plasterers, labourers, and every now and then a queer that comes my way. They're the best fuck, they're so tight. You put some cream on it before you stick it up them and then you slap them on the arse a few times to make them tighter. I must've had more than ten of them, I've lost count.

When Francisco asked him if he had ever been penetrated himself, he replied:

I wouldn't like to feel what those gays feel, it must hurt them. I'm a giver, not a taker. It's not in my book to let someone fuck me.

Not all workers at the site said they had had sexual relations with another man, or took the same attitude towards homosexual behaviour. Some avoided the topic, while others expressed aversion. José Alejandro, for example, said:

I'm not one of your dirt-track riders. I can't stand those bloody queers. I'd like to fry them on a slow fire. I wouldn't do it with a man, because it means seven years bad luck and because what you do to others is what they do to you.

However, it is interesting to note that even those who were most categorical in their refusal to have sexual relations with men made ambivalent comments, even though jokingly. For example, on one occasion when Francisco began to bring up the topic of sex, the previous informant joked: 'Don't tell me we're going to the hotel, because I'll shove your tapeworms back where they came from.' A similar example occurred one night, when Francisco remained behind after work to have a drink with his boss and an estate agent for the condominiums. The latter said he had been to nightclubs where there were transvestites and had even danced with them. 'But I would never dare to screw one of them. I'd rather find a chicken.' So saying he made gestures with his hands to show 'the size of the egg'. The night continued with laughter and toasting: 'to never stop screwing, and never use a condom'.

During the course of the study, Francisco never tried to find out directly whether or not the workers had sexual relations with each other. However, the architects at the site told him they often heard about this kind of thing. They say that when it happens, it is because of alcohol. There may be ceremonies and rituals such as topping out ceremonies which are accompanied by much drinking. One site architect commented:

> At such times that they switch from talk to action. They hit each other, kill each other or have sex. With the alcohol, things work up to a climax. They start touching each other, and the moment comes when, if someone doesn't give in, things can get violent. The next day, you see injuries and you realize what has happened.

Architects also pointed out that they cannot prevent boys of 13 and 14 or even younger from entering the site. These may be among the most vulnerable and those most likely to be used for sex. Consequently, they try to get on the right side of some skilled worker who will protect them.

Among the building workers observed, just over half said they had at some time contracted a sexually transmitted disease. Some mentioned gonorrhoea, others syphilis, while others did not know which.

Subsequent to the investigation, we have had opportunity to cross-check the validity of certain of the comments made by construction workers through interviews with male prostitutes and transvestites. Many of the transvestites interviewed stated that they had had sexual relations with building workers, and some of them even said they were 'the randiest'. One male prostitute stated:

> While there are many who reject you because they have their own lifestyle, there are others who notice you. Sometimes, if you fancy a building worker and go with him, you may even help him out financially. You get no money off a building worker, but you do it for his looks, if you like someone it's all right. Because most of us want something good.

When asked where they got to know the building workers, some explained that when they were working or living near building sites, some of the building workers would follow them or 'chat them up', but the majority said they had met them at neighbourhood *fiestas*, where there are always building workers. A transvestite stated:

> Here you turn up at a *fiesta*, at a neighbourhood party, and there's loads of building workers there. They show their interest in the simplest and most obvious way – they want to dance with you. They show their excitement, their desire for you. They come over and chat to you; it's the looks, the smiles . . . People dressed in women's clothes are the most popular at the dances. Probably because they look absurd or flashy and because some of us dance really well because we get so much practice.

She added:

> We're the best dancers because we have the stamina, because they
> are very strong guys and we can keep going longer than the girls. And
> not just this, but afterwards we don't clear off, we go all the way.

Another transvestite, Paula, talks of her experiences:

> The building workers like our clothes to be very exaggerated. They
> like us to have very painted lips and rouge on the cheeks; this is how
> they envisage cabaret stars, since they are used to looking at porno-
> graphic magazines. They like pornography a lot. Although they can
> see that they're not women, they fancy them.

### Preliminary Conclusions

A building site is a social arena in which there is a vertical and authoritarian,
but informal and unstructured, hierarchy. Through daily interaction between
architects, foremen, skilled workers and labourers, building work is organized.
There are no explicit contracts for the least qualified workers, and no training
centres for the majority of the jobs. Workers learn as they go along. In
construction work, the vertical structure and internal dynamics are sustained
by violence, be it real, threatened or imagined. The person who is at a higher
level constantly has to reaffirm his position. Moreover, working teams are
constantly changed in accordance with the needs of the work. This instability,
and the violence that is generated at work, make it necessary to create ways of
controlling and protecting both human and material resources.

The macho sexual culture shared by the building workers is integrated so
as to organize and control the informal working relationships described
above. The formation, modification and break-up of the working teams are
governed by values and terms specific to the male and female sexual roles,
where the superior is the dominant male and his subordinate is the submissive
female. These sexual roles are maintained through constant verbal and symbolic allusions to copulation whereby the superior achieves and maintains his
position when he manages to penetrate the subordinate metaphorically.
Those who are joined together as if they were man and wife try to apply the
standards that relate to marriage in order to stabilize the relationship and
cope with adversity.

On the building site, besides the constant sexual games, there is constant
talk of sexual adventures. Although the stories of sexual experiences with
other men make up a small part of the repertoire, it may be inferred from the
detailed descriptions offered that many of the workers have engaged in homosexual practices at some time or other. Although it cannot be ruled out that
some of them actively seek such contacts, generally these are of a casual or

circumstantial nature. Sometimes it is just a matter of seizing an unexpected opportunity, such as a chance meeting with a homosexual inclined to permit penetration or with a defenceless young boy, who may even be raped. But building workers boast of these experiences without any shame or modesty. They make it clear that the 'queers' are the others, and refer to them with some contempt, showing that they themselves are just as macho in these relationships as in those they have with women. In their opinion, such actions bring out their characteristics of maleness and dominance.

The patterns of bisexual behaviour described here are central to Mexican culture. They share features in common with the kinds of bisexuality described by Cáceres in Peru, Shifter in Costa Rica and Parker in Brazil elsewhere in this book. Because of their possible implications for HIV transmission, there is a need for more study of such practices in different social and working environments. Processes such as seasonal migration, when the migrant goes in search of work, most usually without his family, may be particularly conducive to the homosexual practices referred to. Mexican workers who emigrate to the United States, for example, take their own culture and values with them, and the majority continue to spend their time with their fellow countrymen or other Latin Americans often in isolated and difficult circumstances. Their likelihood of acquiring HIV infection cannot therefore be analysed solely on the basis of whether or not they come into contact with a population which already has higher infection rates, but depends on many factors including those internal to working groups. The same is true of internal migration within Mexico.

### Intervention Implications

*Siendo agujero aunque sea de caballero.* (Refrán popular)[11]

In Mexico, several obstacles confront health promotion about HIV and AIDS. The patterns of bisexuality described here imply the need to develop strategies for three different, but related parties, with different levels of risk: men who identify themselves as homosexual or gay, men who define themselves as heterosexual but who are occasionally (or regularly) homosexually active, and the female partners of men who are bisexually active.

In order to be effective, interventions will need to address different levels of biological and social vulnerability, different levels of risk awareness, and different likelihoods of influencing risk behaviour. With respect to risk behaviour, it has been widely documented that unprotected receptive anal sex carries the highest risk of infection, followed by unprotected vaginal sex, and unprotected insertive anal or vaginal sex. With respect to risk awareness, those who are currently in the most favourable position are probably men who identify themselves as homosexual, and who have regular contact with gay or AIDS organizations and/or the commercial gay scene. Partly as a result of grassroots community action, and partly as a result of tabloid press sensationalism, their risk awareness is likely to be higher than those of other groups, particularly men who do not see their sexual behaviour with other men as homosexual or bisexual, and women in monogamous relationships who do not know, or do not want to know, what their husbands or regular partners are doing. But even among those whose risk awareness may be high, behaviour change may be difficult to achieve as recent research in Mexico among men who see themselves as homosexual or gay has shown (Ramírez *et al.*, 1994).

The promotion of condoms has come up against huge barriers in Mexico. Some of these derive from the conservatism of people at large, for whom condom use may be difficult to discuss. Others derive from moral barriers and the economic influence that the conservative right holds over the media. Within such a context, to talk of male infidelity is difficult, and to talk about male infidelity with other men unthinkable. Those who are in the worst position are probably women because, even if they possess an awareness of risk, they lack the social power to protect themselves. For many, their only risk behaviour is having sex with their husband or regular partner. It is still difficult to conceive of practical health promotion interventions for such women that would significantly reduce their vulnerability to HIV and AIDS.

Turning now to intervention efforts among the men whose lives have been described in this chapter. In 1992, following efforts to sensitize the National Chamber of Construction to the potential impact that HIV and AIDS could have on the construction industry workforce, a meeting took place between representatives of their training department and trainers based in CONASIDA. During the course of these initial discussions, construction industry representatives acknowledged the existence of many of the behaviours and lifestyles described here. This initial meeting led to subsequent training workshops and the development of educational resources for distribution among construction industry workers. It also enabled a team from CONASIDA to visit twenty-five construction sites through which they reached 1,800 builders. On these visits, great interest was shown by the workers. It is planned that such work should continue, and the experience gained may be extended to other trades or professions organized in a similar way, perhaps through one or more national trade unions.

In the medium to longer term, such health promotion efforts with construction industry workers will need to be complemented by other initiatives involving their prospective or potential sexual partners, including homosexual and gay men, as well as male and female sex workers. Given present relatively low levels of reported condom use, condom promotion should be central within such efforts, utilizing perhaps the not inconsiderable resources and marketing power of condom manufacturers themselves.

## Concluding Comments

*Caras vemos, corazones no sabemos.* (Refrán popular)[12]

In Mexico in the field of AIDS, the predominant cultural climate on sexuality and morality poses major difficulties for educational intervention by governmental and non-governmental groups, and puts obstacles in the way of public health interventions in the area of HIV prevention. The powerful influence of the Catholic church, and its links with business groups, have held back more determined health promotion efforts, leaving gaps in provision that are truly criminal.

It is essential that in future efforts the Mexican state puts the interest of public health before the ideology of conservative forces which try to reduce AIDS to questions of morality. But progressive forces have great challenges to face. It is urgent that they should achieve legitimacy for a new cultural agenda that questions double standards of morality, accepts female sexuality and recognizes the sexual behaviour and love of those who are outside heterosexual 'normality'. Homophobia creates an atmosphere in which people who have homosexual desires will not act upon them consciously or deliberately. So long as this does not change, there will be a growing number of cases of HIV among 'heterosexual' men who have sex with other men, and their female partners. Such individual and social denial is compounded by the overall national political atmosphere, the absence of a strong gay movement and scant effort by political parties and public figures to challenge and criticize homophobia. There is still much to do, therefore, to stimulate debate about the right to be different. And with regard to the public health, more effective health promotion interventions to combat AIDS must be made a priority. They cannot be delayed any longer.

## Notes

1 The authors would like to thank Linda Alcaraz who assisted in the translation of various parts of this chapter.
2 Translation: 'What's the difference between a Mexican who is homosexual, and one who is not? Two drinks!' Joke told in Mexico.
3 A *pulquería* is a type of bar that only sells pulque, a very cheap alcoholic beverage with a low alcohol content.
4 Translation: 'Who is completely heterosexual? Nobody. Isn't that the truth?'
5 Translation: 'Any hole [will do], even if it belongs to a chicken' (popular saying).
6 Other writers do not agree that *mayates* only have sexual relations with other men for material gain. In general, a man is called a *mayate* if, having identified himself as heterosexual as well as having sexual relations

with women, he has them with men (Hernández J. C., 1994; Prieur, 1994).

7 Other authors use the term *buga* to talk about men who are strictly heterosexual. There also exists a word *chacal* to describe heterosexual men who make fun of homosexuals, but who may have sexual relationships with them when very 'drunk'.

8 The title of the video makes reference to different flavours of *tamales*, a typical Mexican dish made from maize flour wrapped in maize or banana leaves and steamed. It offers a good metaphor for the idea of bisexuality.

9 Translation: 'With a good-looking builder, we girls say, well if you've had a nice bath well I'll go for it, but if it comes to it, with a bit of wine we can forget the bath altogether.'

10 All the workers' names are fictitious.

11 Translation: 'Any hole [is all right] even if it belongs to a gentleman' (popular saying).

12 Translation: 'We can see faces, but we can't know hearts' (populr saying).

## References

*Boletín Mensual SIDA/ETS*, año 8, núm. 11, nov. de 1994, INDRE, México. 2782.

Carrier, J. M. (1976a) 'Cultural Factors Affecting Urban Mexican Male Homosexual Behavior', *Archives of Sexual Behavior*, 5, 2, pp. 103–24.

Carrier, J. M. (1976b) 'Family Attitudes and Mexican Male Homosexuality', *Urban Life*, 5, 359–75.

Carrier, J. M. (1985) 'Mexican Male Bisexuality', in Klein, F. and Wolf, T. J. (Eds) *Bisexualities: Theory and Research*, New York, Haworth Press.

Carrier, J. M. (1989a) 'Sexual Behavior and Spread of AIDS in México', *Medical Anthropology*, 10, pp. 129–42.

Carrier, J. M. (1989b) 'Gay Liberation and Coming Out in Mexico', *Gay and Lesbian Youth*, New York, Haworth Press.

Carrier, J. M. and Magaña, R. (1991) 'Use of Ethnosexual Data on Men of Mexican Origin for HIV/AIDS Prevention Program', *Journal of Sex Research*, 28, 2, pp. 189–202.

CONASIDA (1994) *Comportamiento sexual en la cuidad de México. Encuesta 1992–1993*, CONASIDA, 203.

García, M., Valdespino, J. A., Izazola, J., Palacios, M. and Sepúlveda, J. (1991) 'Bisexuality in Mexico: Current Perspectives', in Tielman, R. A. P., Carballo, M. and Hendriks, A. C. (Eds) *Bisexuality and HIV/AIDS*, Buffalo, NY, Prometheus.

González Block, M. A. and Liguori, A. L. (1992) *El SIDA en los estratos socioeconómicos de México*, Instituto Nacional de Salud Pública, Serie Perspectivas en Salud Pública.

Hernández, J. C. (1994) 'Homofobia: causa de prácticas sexuales de alto riesgo en la adolescencia y juventud temprana', proyecto en manuscrito.

HERNÁNDEZ, M., URIBE, P., GORTMAKER, S., AVILA, C., DE CASO, L. E., MULLER, N. and SEPÚLVEDA, J. (1992) 'Sexual Behavior and Status for Human Immunodeficiency Virus Type 1 Among Homosexual and Bisexual Males in Mexico City', *American Journal of Epidemiology*, 135, 8, pp. 883–94.

IZAZOLA, J. A. (1994) 'La Bisexualidad', in PORRÚA, M. A. (Ed.) *Antología Sobre Sexualidad Humana*, tomo 1' México.

IZAZOLA, J. A., VALDESPINO, J. L. and SEPÚLVEDA, J. (1988) 'Factores de riesgo asociados a infección pro VIH en hombres homosexuales y bisexuales', *Salud Pública*, 30, 4.

IZAZOLA, J. A., VALDESPINO, J. L., GORTMAKER, S. L., TOWNSEND, J., BECKER, J., PALACIOS, M., MULLER, N. and SEPÚLVEDA, J. (1991) 'HIV Seropositivity and Behavioral and Sociological Risks among Homosexual and Bisexual Men in Six Mexican Cities', *Journal of Acquired Immune Deficiency Syndromes*, 4, 614–22.

LEÑERO, V. (1964) *Los albañiles*, México, Seix Barral.

LUMSDEN, I. (1991) *Homosexuality, Society and the State in Mexico*, México, Canadian Gay Archives y Solediciones.

MAGAÑA, J. R. and CARRIER, J. M. (1991) 'Mexican and Mexican American Male Sexual Behavior and Spread of AIDS in California', *Journal of Sex Research*, 28, 3, pp. 426–41.

PAZ, O. (1950) *El laberinto de la soledad*, Mexico, Fondo de Cultura Económica.

PRIEUR, A. (1994a) 'Power and Pleasure: Male Homosexuality and the Construction of Masculinity in Mexico', presentation at 48th International Congress of Americanists, Stockholm/Uppsala.

PRIEUR, A. (1994b) 'I Am My Own Special Creation: Mexican Homosexual Transvestites' Construction of Femininity', *Young-Nordic Journal of Youth Research*, 2, 2, p. 16.

RAMÍREZ, J., SUÁREZ, E., DE LA ROSA, G., CASTRO, M. A. and ZIMMERMAN, M. A. (1994) 'AIDS Knowledge and Sexual Behavior Among Mexican Gay and Bisexual Men', *AIDS Education and Prevention*, 6, 2, pp. 163–74.

RAMÍREZ HEREDIA, R. (1984) 'El Rayo Macoy', in MORTIZ, JOAQUÍN (Ed.) *El Rayo Macoy*, México.

SECRETARÍA DE SALUD (1988) 'Hombres homo-bisexuales', in *Informe técnico. Evaluación del Impacto de la estragia educativa para la prevención del SIDA: México 1987–88*, Secretaría de Salud y Population Council.

ZAPATA, L. (1979) *El vampiro de la colonia Roma*, Mexico, Grijalbo.

## Chapter 6

# Bisexual Communities and Cultures in Costa Rica

*Jacobo Schifter and Johnny Madrigal*
*with Peter Aggleton*

Costa Rica is a small Central American nation, comprising an area of 50,000 square kilometres and with a population of 3 million people. The country is comprised of people of Spanish descent, since most of the native Indian population was decimated during colonial times. The nation has the longest history of democratic government in Latin America and abolished its army in 1948. Its main sources of income are tourism, coffee and banana exports. Notwithstanding the fact that it is a developing country, Costa Rica has a large middle class.

By 1994 there had been 644 reported cases of AIDS in Costa Rica. For the last three years, behaviourally homosexual men have been the group most affected by the epidemic (they currently make up 55 per cent of accumulated cases). According to 1994 data, 17 per cent of the total of cases of the syndrome in the country were behaviourally bisexual men. The study of bisexuality is therefore of vital importance to an understanding of HIV transmission. Knowledge of the cultural aspects of bisexuality, and of its relationship to the epidemic, will help the planning and implementation of information and education campaigns to prevent new infections.

## Questions of Definition

Some authors adhere to the thesis that the bisexual individual is someone who has sexual contact with men and women. This thesis, shared by Churchill (1967), Ford and Beach (1951) and Kinsey *et al.* (1948), defines bisexuality as a sexual practice. Other researchers consider that bisexual individuals possess characteristics which cannot be defined simply in terms of sexual practice. Among the criteria to be considered are desire, the degree of attraction felt toward persons of both sexes (Blumstein and Schwartz, 1976a, 1976b; Klein, 1978) and self-definition, the individual's definition of his or her sexual identity (Warren, 1974). Still others believe that bisexuality should be defined more in terms of 'dual affective preference', the desire to have close and enduring relationships with men and women, and that sexual contact should not be the determining factor (MacInnes, 1973; Bode, 1976; Klein, 1978; Scott, 1978). Klein (1980) offers a complex model for bisexuality that takes account not only of attraction and sexual experience, but also sexual fantasies, emotional and social preferences, self-definition, and the homosexual or bisexual lifestyle of the individual.

The above models fail to take into account differing cultural interpretations of sexual behaviour. Different sexual communities might give varying interpretations to similar sexual acts. As we will show later, one sexual culture may understand bisexual practice as a different sexual orientation, whereas another may see it as part of the heterosexual norm. Part of the definition of who the bisexual is, therefore, is a cultural and social prerogative. Attention to variations in sexual practice, desire, self-definition and cultural interpretation is therefore essential in making sense of the lives of men who have sex with men and women in Costa Rica.

### Patterns of Bisexuality

There are several groups of men who feel desire for both women and men, and have bisexual practices. Most of them do not feel they belong to any group other than the heterosexual majority, nor do they perceive themselves as possessing a different sexual orientation. Carrier (1985) in his study in Mexico argued that bisexual practice does not link in any direct way to having a different sexual orientation. He advanced the idea that for many Mexican youths, having sexual relations with effeminate boys was culturally acceptable. The boys who were active in anal sex were not considered either homosexual or bisexual. Since society did not stigmatize the practice, a conscious awareness of having a bisexual orientation does not arise.

A similar group of men, known as *cacheros*, exists in Costa Rica. These are men who are practising bisexuals but who are neither perceived as such by others, nor so defined by themselves. *Cacheros* are masculine-looking men who are 'officially' the penetrators in anal sex. They may also have sexual relations with women. Here we will focus on two different groups of *cacheros*: those in prison and those who are the regular lovers of transvestites.

*Cacheros* are, however, not the only men who practise bisexuality without claimimg such an identity. There are other groups who are also practising bisexuals and do not define themselves as such. These include married homosexual men pressured into marriage to avoid discrimination, and *chulos* or male sex workers who have sex for money.

In Costa Rica today there is also a small group of single and married men who do define themselves as bisexual and are thus perceived by others. This sector is numerically the smallest and the most difficult to make contact with. As opposed to *chulos* and *cacheros*, self-identified bisexuals are not concentrated in any sector of the city, nor is their activity institutionalized as in prison. They also do not often socialize in gay bars. Nevertheless, such men do have sexual relations with more exclusively homosexual men, and those reported on here were identified through that avenue.

In this chapter, we will look at the HIV/AIDS-related beliefs and behaviour of self-identified bisexuals compared with those who are homosexual in their identity. We will also analyse the same variables for two different groups of *cachero* men: prisoners, and lovers of transvestites. We hope to show how social factors such as prostitution, incarceration and drugs have an impact on identity, sexual practice and risks of HIV infection.

### Study Methods

#### Self-Defined Bisexuals

The principal source of information used in researching self-identified bisexuals was a study on AIDS-related knowledge, sexual behaviour and sexual culture among bisexuals and homosexual males undertaken in 1989–90 with the financial support and technical assisstance of the then Social and Behavioral Research Unit of the World Health Organization (WHO) Global Programme on AIDS (GPA). A questionnaire was given to 443 men who have sex with men, of whom a quota were self-identified bisexual men.

#### Men Who Have Sex in Prison

Four sources of information were used to shed light on sexual relations between men in La Reforma, the largest prison in Costa Rica. These included two-hour in-depth interviews with eight openly homosexual men in prison conducted between October 1989 and January 1990; data from a questionnaire which was distributed to twenty-two openly homosexual men in prison in February 1990; data from forty-five in-depth interviews conducted with prison personnel in January 1990; and data collected in weekly focus groups carried out with fifteen openly homosexual men in prison between March and June 1990.

#### Men Who Are Lovers of Transvestites

In 1990, an ethnographic study and in-depth interviews, as well as a survey of attitudes and knowledge of AIDS, was carried out among the transvestite population of the red light district in San José. Transvestites and their lovers were also visited in their homes throughout different areas of the city. Over a three-month period, twenty-two closed-ended interviews and twenty in-depth interviews were carried out (Shifter and Madrigal, 1992).

### Self-Identified Bisexuals

Two methods were used to obtain a sample of self-identified bisexual men. First, interviewers were asked to contact bisexual friends and acquaintances in order to establish the quota required in the aforementioned WHO study of men who have sex with men. Second, when the data from the 443 questionnaires of men who have sex with men were analysed, further behaviourally bisexual men were selected on the basis of their responses to selected items on the sexual attraction and practice scales. The working definition of bisexuality used to select the sample was 'an individual who currently has attraction for, and has sex with, persons of both sexes'. From a total of 443 who have sex with men, sixty were classified as bisexuals (scoring 2, 3 or 4 on the scale). For purposes of comparison, a group of exclusively homosexual men was also constituted (value 5 on the scale). This exclusively homosexual group totalled 215.

### Definition and Evolution in Time

In fact, not all the men who were labelled as bisexuals by interviewers turned out to be so according to our definition. The interviewers had identified fifty-two men as bisexuals but 17 per cent of them did not fit our definition. A further fifty-nine defined themselves bisexuals but the interviewers did not agree with them.

Bisexuality is not only affected by people's definitions, but also by time. Klein (1980) considers that bisexuality or homosexuality should not be seen as static categories, but rather that these change over time. Data here confirm his thesis. Of the bisexuals studied, only 62 per cent had sexual relations with males and females five years previously, and 17 per cent did so ten years previously. Exclusive heterosexual behaviour diminishes over time among bisexuals, concomitant with an increase in their homosexual behaviour. Homosexuals, on the other hand, show a more stable pattern, since 80 per cent had sex with males five years previously, and 57 per cent did so ten years previously (see Table 6.1). In their studies of bisexuality, MacInnes (1973) and Money (1980) state that bisexuality is rarely characterized by symmetrical sexual attraction and practices with males and females. Data here seem to confirm this view. Only 20 per cent of the bisexuals stated that they had the same amount of sexual activity with males and females at present, and only 27 per cent felt equally attracted towards both sexes.

### Marital Status

A key feature of bisexual practice is marital status, given the danger of HIV transmission. Only a quarter of the bisexuals studied were cohabiting or

*Table 6.1 Bisexuals and Homosexuals: Change in Sexual Orientation Over Time by Sexual Practice and Attraction* (percentages of 52 bisexuals and 215 homosexuals)

| Sexual Practice and Attraction Scale | Bisexuals | | | Homosexuals | | |
|---|---|---|---|---|---|---|
| | Now | 5 years ago | 10 years ago | Now | 5 years ago | 10 years ago |
| **Sexual Practice** | | | | | | |
| 1 | – | 21 | 35 | – | 1 | 2 |
| 2 | 37 | 27 | 7 | – | 1 | 1 |
| 3 | 20 | 13 | 3 | – | 1 | 2 |
| 4 | 43 | 22 | 7 | – | 7 | 4 |
| 5 | – | 10 | 12 | 100 | 80 | 57 |
| 6 | – | 7 | 37 | – | 10 | 34 |
| **Attraction** | | | | | | |
| 1 | – | 13 | 35 | – | 1 | 2 |
| 2 | 35 | 28 | 8 | – | 1 | 3 |
| 3 | 27 | 23 | 18 | – | 2 | 2 |
| 4 | 38 | 28 | 17 | – | 8 | 8 |
| 5 | – | 7 | 7 | 100 | 82 | 65 |
| 6 | – | – | 15 | – | 6 | 20 |

married. Additional data, not reported on here, suggest that the majority of the bisexuals studied did not have a stable relationship with a woman.

### Sexual Activity

The average number of sexual partners during the last twelve months for bisexuals was 17.2 males and 8.5 females (see Table 6.2). Men who were exclusively homosexual reported having a higher average number of male partners (28.7), and a lower average of female partners (0.1).

### Knowledge of AIDS

Both groups possessed substantial knowledge of the ways HIV is transmitted, and there were no significant differences between them. Ninety-eight per cent of the bisexuals and 96 per cent of the homosexuals were aware that HIV can be transmitted by semen. Ninety-five per cent of both groups were also aware that it can be transmitted by blood, and 88 per cent and 90 per cent respectively knew that a condom serves as a barrier against the virus (Table 6.3). In

*Table 6.2 Male and Female Sexual Partners of Bisexuals and Homosexuals during the Last Twelve Months and the Last Thirty Days*

| Partners | Bisexuals | | Homosexuals | |
|---|---|---|---|---|
| | Males | Females | Males | Females |
| Number interviewed | 60 | | 215 | |
| In last 12 months | | | | |
| Average | 17.2 | 8.5 | 28.7 | 0.1 |
| Mode | 1 | 1 | 1 | 0 |
| Median | 3 | 1 | 5 | 0 |
| Lowest | 0 | 0 | 0 | 0 |
| Highest | 200 | 100 | 1000 | 8 |
| In last 30 days | | | | |
| Average | 2.3 | 1.0 | 2.9 | 0.01 |
| Mode | 1 | 0 | 1 | 0 |
| Median | 1 | 1 | 1 | 0 |
| Lowest | 0 | 1 | 0 | 0 |
| Highest | 20 | 10 | 103 | 3 |

spite of this knowledge, one-fifth of the respondents participated in non-monogamous sexual intercourse without the protection of a condom. This leads us to conclude that extensive HIV-related knowledge does not explain (or guarantee) safe sexual practices.

### Attitudes towards and Use of Condoms

Bisexuals as well as homosexuals stated that they used condoms regularly. Slightly more than half of the respondents stated that they always used one. Approximately one-quarter of those interviewed used one occasionally, and one-fifth said they either do not currently use one or have never used one. In order to assess the veracity of the information provided by the respondents, they were asked about their sexual practices without a condom during the last thirty days. The results show, among other things, that of the bisexuals who asserted that they always used a condom, 21 per cent reported having had sexual intercourse with a female without using protection, and in the case of the homosexuals, 9 per cent reported having had passive anal sex without using a condom (Table 6.3). These results suggest that, in reality, the percentage always using a condom is even lower. Making the necessary adjustments, it can be estimated that less than half (43 per cent) of the bisexuals, and 47 per cent of the homosexuals, always used

*Table 6.3 Bisexuals and Homosexuals: Percentage with Correct Responses to Questions Concerning HIV Transmission and Safer Sex*

| Transmission and prevention | Bisexuals | Homosexuals |
|---|---|---|
| Number of men interviewed | 60 | 215 |
| Percentage correct responses | | |
| Transmitted through semen | 98 | 96 |
| Transmitted through blood | 95 | 95 |
| Due to the long incubation period it might be transmitted by a seemingly healthy person | 93 | 91 |
| Condom use prevents infection | 88 | 90 |
| Condom use frequency: percentage of respondents | | |
| Always | 55 | 52 |
| Almost always | 16 | 10 |
| Sometimes | 8 | 11 |
| Hardly ever | 1 | 6 |
| Never now | 2 | 5 |
| Never has used | 17 | 16 |
| Penetration without a condom during last month: percentage of respondents | | |
| Female – anal | 6 | 0 |
| Female – vaginal | 21 | 0.9 |
| Male – insertive | 6 | 9 |
| Male – receptive | 9 | 5 |
| Percentage of respondents at high risk of acquiring HIV during last 30 days | 25 | 18 |

a condom in their sexual activities, and that close to one-third used one occasionally.

### Unsafe Sexual Practices

In order to examine unsafe sexual practices in both groups, we calculated the percentage of respondents who had had anal or vaginal sex without a condom during the last six months, and during the thirty days prior to interview. As can be seen in Table 6.3, there is a great deal of unprotected sexual activity. In the case of bisexual respondents, 50 per cent had had vaginal intercourse without a condom at least once during the previous six months, and 43 per cent had engaged in insertive anal sex with men during the same period and under the same conditions. During the same time period, 35 per cent of the homosexuals had had unprotected insertive anal sex with men, and 40 per cent had had unprotected receptive anal sex.

### Perceived Risk of Infection

Among the bisexuals, the results obtained indicate that those who consider vaginal sex and insertive and receptive anal penetration without a condom to be high-risk practices tend to have, in relative terms, significantly lower levels of this type of behaviour (see Table 6.4). This suggests that those who perceive correctly the risk in these unsafe sexual practices tend to avoid them more than those who do not.

### Attitudes towards Condoms and Unsafe Sex

One of the factors that could influence an individual's unsafe sexual behaviour is his attitudes toward condoms. Table 6.5 shows that a majority of those participating in unsafe sexual practices do not like condoms, and that those with safer practices tend to have a more positive attitude in this respect. Tests of association show that among both bisexuals and homosexuals, unsafe sexual practices with male partners are associated with negative attitudes towards the condom. There is no association, however, between attitudes and unsafe sex on the part of bisexuals in their sexual practices with women.

*Table 6.4 Bisexuals and Homosexuals: Risk-Perception of Vaginal, Active Anal and Passive Anal Penetration without Condom, and Sexual Practice during the Last Thirty Days (percentages)*

| Practised activity in the last 30 days | Perception of risk of infection | Total | (n) | Bisexuals | | (n) | Homosexuals | |
|---|---|---|---|---|---|---|---|---|
| | | | | Yes | No | | Yes | No |
| | Vaginal penetration without condom | | | (0.02)** | | | (0.89) | |
| Low | | 100 | 31 | 68 | 32 | 115 | 99 | 1 |
| High | | 100 | 29 | 93 | 7 | 100 | 99 | 1 |
| | Active penetration without condom | | | (0.007)* | | | (0.3) | |
| Low | | 100 | 16 | 50 | 50 | 47 | 75 | 25 |
| High | | 100 | 44 | 84 | 16 | 167 | 81 | 19 |
| | Passive penetration without condom | | | (0.05)** | | | (0.0001)* | |
| Low | | 100 | 14 | 100 | – | 35 | 51 | 49 |
| High | | 100 | 46 | 77 | 23 | 180 | 83 | 17 |

*Note*: The parentheses include the significant $\chi^2$ values for the total of 60 bisexuals and 215 homosexuals.

*significant at 0.0001.

**significant at 0.05.

*Table 6.5 Unsafe Sexual Practices among Bisexuals and Homosexuals during the Last Thirty Days and Attitudes Toward Condoms*

| Sexual orientation and practice | Total | Diminishes sexual pleasure | | Makes one lose concentration | |
|---|---|---|---|---|---|
| | | Agree | Disagree | Agree | Disagree |
| **Bisexuals** | | | | | |
| Vaginal penetration without condom | | (0.88) | | (0.01)** | |
| Yes | 100 | 46 | 54 | 32 | 68 |
| No | 100 | 48 | 52 | 67 | 33 |
| Active anal penetration without condom | | (0.004)* | | (0.08)*** | |
| Yes | 100 | 71 | 29 | 64 | 36 |
| No | 100 | 31 | 69 | 39 | 61 |
| Passive anal penetration without condom | | (0.002)* | | (0.03)** | |
| Yes | 100 | 100 | – | 80 | 20 |
| No | 100 | 35 | 65 | 42 | 58 |
| **Homosexuals** | | | | | |
| Vaginal penetration without condom | | (0.56) | | (0.61) | |
| Yes | 100 | 33 | 67 | 60 | 40 |
| No | 100 | 45 | 55 | 48 | 52 |
| Active anal penetration without condom | | (0.000)* | | (0.02)** | |
| Yes | 100 | 66 | 34 | 60 | 40 |
| No | 100 | 35 | 65 | 43 | 57 |
| Passive anal penetration without condom | | (0.006)* | | (0.03)** | |
| Yes | 100 | 58 | 42 | 59 | 41 |
| No | 100 | 38 | 62 | 43 | 57 |

*Note*: The parentheses include the significant $\chi^2$ values for a total of 60 bisexuals and 215 homosexuals.

*significant at 0.001.
**significant at 0.05.
***significant at 0.1.

### Drug Use and Unsafe Sex

The questionnaire elicited information on the frequency of use of different drugs during the last six months, before and during intercourse. Respondents were also asked whether they had participated or not in specific sexual practices, with both males and females, and without using a condom. This provides

Table 6.6 *Unsafe Sexual Practices among Bisexuals and Homosexuals during the Last Six Months, and its Relation to Drug Use ($\chi^2$ Significant Values)*

| Sexual practice without using condom | Drug use before or during sex | | | | | |
|---|---|---|---|---|---|---|
| | Alcohol | | Marijuana | | Cocaine | |
| | Before | During | Before | During | Before | During |
| **Bisexuals** | | | | | | |
| Number Interviewed | 39 | | 18 | | 9 | |
| Vaginal penetration | 0.09** | 0.21 | 0.22 | 0.54 | 0.69 | 0.40 |
| Insertive penetration | 0.48 | 0.45 | 0.16 | 0.87 | 0.23 | 0.36 |
| Receptive penetration | 0.32 | 0.65 | 0.04* | 0.21 | 0.32 | 0.60 |
| **Homosexuals** | | | | | | |
| Number Interviewed | 145 | | 48 | | 21 | |
| Vaginal penetration | 0.49 | 0.02* | – | – | – | – |
| Insertive penetration | 0.14 | 0.54 | 0.58 | 0.67 | 0.18 | 0.54 |
| Receptive penetration | 0.39 | 0.06** | 0.71 | 0.84 | 0.01* | 0.23 |

*Note*: Penetration without condom was classified under 'Yes' or 'No'. Drug use before or during sex was recoded as 'Never', 'Almost never' or 'Rarely' and 'Always' and 'Almost always.'

*Values significant to 0.05.
**Values significant to 0.1.

useful information to ascertain whether the frequency of use of a specific drug is related to specific types of sexual activity.

With regard to bisexual men who indicated having consumed alcohol prior to or during sexual intercourse with women, a positive correlation was found between the frequency of alcohol consumption before having sex and unprotected vaginal sex. A positive correlation was also found between marijuana use before and during sex with a man, and engaging in unprotected receptive anal sex (see Table 6.6).

### Sexual Culture in Prison

Homosexual behaviour in prisons is as old as the penitentiary system itself. Ellis (1905/1936) in his famous *Studies in the Psychology of Sex*, says that approximately 80 per cent of men are sexually perverse, although he emphasizes that in 'moments of pessimism he believes that in reality they all are'. Fishman (1951) in the classic book *Sex Practices of Prisoners*, first published in 1934, claims that the percentage of North American prisoners who practise homosexuality varied between 30 and 40 per cent at that time.

From our in-depth interviews, it became evident that between 70 and 90 per cent of the inmates have homosexual relationships. Those interviewed reported having had an average of 51 sexual partners during the past 6 months. One of them reported having had sex with 365 different partners. Prison officials also report high percentages. Based on the ethnographic information we can identify various types of homosexual relations in prison:

1 The *cachero* (topman) and the transvestite – the *cachero* is the masculine man who is supposedly the anal penetrator in a homosexual relationship;
2 The older man and the *cabrito* (chicken) – the *cabrito* is a young, often beardless adolescent. The older man provides him with money and protection; the sexual practice varies;
3 Two closet homosexuals (called *zorras*, or possums, in Costa Rica). This relationship is based less on power and more in mutual reciprocity.

Although these are steady relationships involving sexual intercourse, members of a relationship also have occasional contacts with other inmates.

In many ways the Greek concept of pederasty may be more useful in making sense of prison culture and the kind of human relationships that emerge in this context than modern Western ideas about sexual orientation. According to Halperin (1990), the ancient Greeks defined sexuality not in terms of the object of desire but in the terms of an active-passive dichotomy. Free men and citizens of Greece were those who were the penetrators in their relations with women, slaves, youths and foreigners. In prison in Costa Rica, the Greek model is still prevalent, with some modifications. Broadly speaking, men can be divided into those who are active (insertive) and those who are passive (receptive) and homosexual relations are accepted only between these two groups. It is not accepted (even though it sometimes happens) for two masculine or two effeminate men to get together. A too-young *cachero* is not respected by older men and may be raped to show him that he should not mess with transvestites or other effeminate men. When youths get older in prison, however, they are expected to become *cacheros* themselves.

But differing from the Greeks, it is not sexual practice that determines who is a *cachero* in jail but his power as a gang leader or as a dangerous and violent man. While the *cachero* can experiment sexually and be anally penetrated by a transvestite or a youth, he is still a *cachero* because he is the one with the capacity to kill. No one dares to question his masculinity by reason of these variations in his sexual behaviour. He is not defined as a homosexual.

### Use of the Condom

The majority of sexual acts in prison do not involve the use of a condom. Forty-one per cent of respondents reported not using condoms, 37 per cent of those interviewed used them occasionally and only 23 per cent reported using them

Table 6.7 *Prisoners: Frequency of Condom Use*

| Frequency of use | Number of transvestites | Percentage |
|---|---|---|
| Total | 22 | 100 |
| Frequency | | |
| Always | 5 | 23 |
| Almost always | 3 | 14 |
| Sometimes | 3 | 14 |
| Almost never | 2 | 9 |
| Never | 4 | 18 |
| Never used it | 5 | 23 |

Table 6.8 *Prisoners: Unprotected Insertive and Receptive Anal Sex*

| Period of reference | Anal penetration without condom use | | | |
|---|---|---|---|---|
| | Insertive | | Receptive | |
| | (N) | (%) | (N) | (%) |
| Total | 22 | 100 | 22 | 100 |
| Last 6 months | | | | |
| Yes | 12 | 54 | 16 | 73 |
| No | 10 | 46 | 6 | 27 |

always (see Table 6.7), a somewhat high figure in view of the poor availability of condoms in prison.

Just over half of those interviewed had anally penetrated another man without using a condom during the past six months, and nearly three-quarters reported having been anally penetrated without a condom during this same time period (see Table 6.8). These figures should however be treated as conservative estimates of risk. During the course of fieldwork, it was observed that the frequency of reported sexual encounters was greater than the number indicated in the questionnaire.

### Knowledge about AIDS

Although AIDS was first identified in 1981, inmates at La Reforma heard about it much later. Fifty per cent were not aware of it until 1985 or later. The majority of those interviewed knew the main forms of transmission and prevention and, to a lesser degree, the symptoms of infection. Considering that there is a high level of knowledge about AIDS transmission and prevention, and condom use is low, it can be deduced that there are more important factors determining the use of condoms.

### Rules of the Game in Relationships

Prison culture is filled with contradictions. There is tolerance towards homosexuality among the inmates and an aggressive masculine culture, alongside a hostility towards the weak and feminine. In order to survive, the inmate must learn to defend himself and take care of his space. For this reason, physical strength and having sharp weapons is indispensable. In a prison culture that places a high value on masculinity, homosexual relations are tolerated as long as sexual roles are respected. A feminine and weak person can establish a relation with a *cachero*, that is, a man that is masculine and not officially defined as a homosexual. The first one presents himself socially as a woman and the second as a man. To maintain the separate roles, the 'homosexual', or the transvestite, always uses a woman's name, dresses like a woman and does 'women's work' for the *cachero*: ironing, washing, cleaning. When speaking about his lover with others, the *cachero* always refers to the transvestite with the pronoun 'she'. In this relationship, the *cachero* provides protection for his lover, preventing the latter from being accosted by other men.

Another type of relationship tolerated by prison culture is between an older man and a younger man or *cabrito*. Adolescent inmates are sought by long-term inmates who are looking for a controlling relationship. They seek 'feminine' services in exchange for protecting the young man in the penitentiary. Although in this type of relationship there is no marked gender difference, the age difference allows the older man to see himself as 'macho' and protect the younger or weaker one.

*Cacheros*, however, also engage in sexual relations with their wives, female friends and lovers during conjugal visits and weekend visits and when they are on leave from the prison. For example, C, a *cachero* who is the lover of R, a transvestite, has sexual relations with R's sister and cousin (who is a sex worker) at the same time when they visit at the weekends. To prevent R from getting jealous, C has sexual relations with him, having had intercourse with the sister the same day.

Sexism is an element of culture which encourages multiple contacts. In penal cultures, *cacheros* must not be sexually faithful to transvestites. For this reason, they seduce other transvestites, like a Don Juan who has more than one woman. Several of them also have sexual relations with closet homosexuals or *zorras*. A *cachero* therefore maintains relations with various men and 'women' at the same time in the penitentiary.

### Hierarchy

In a prison, as in a patriarchal society, there is a clearly established hierarchy. The transvestite is under the control of the *cachero*. The constant threats of the *cachero* hang over her daily existence. A scene of jealousy between a couple could easily turn into a knife fight. Nearly all the transvestites interviewed have scars resulting from fights with the other inmates. Because they assume the role of the 'woman' in the couple's relationship, transvestites are trapped in the same obligations and enjoy as few rights as women have in Latin American society.

In the course of fieldwork in prisons, transvestites said they have had great problems trying to convince lovers to use condoms for anal sex. If they suggest using condoms, *cacheros* become suspicious of their health or their fidelity. For the *cachero*'s macho image, infidelity is an affront, endangering his reputation. When transvestites engage in prostitution, it must be done surreptitiously.

The little power that the transvestite has in the role he assumes in the relationship makes it difficult to use condoms. Fifty-eight per cent of those interviewed indicated that it was the attitude of their partner that determined use.

### Prostitution

The transvestite in a relationship becomes the provider, an ironic position in the prison given that he supposedly is playing the role of the 'woman'. Some earn money by doing domestic work for the rest of the inmates: they wash or iron clothes. Others have raffles, selling numbers in combination with the national lottery. But in a system with few work opportunities, transvestites are even harder to place in work positions. Almost all consider industrial or agricultural work very hard. In order to satisfy their own needs and those of other inmates, they resort to prostitution. This activity is often hidden from their lover for fear of retribution.

During the course of fieldwork, transvestites indicated several times that the problem with using condoms is that paying partners do not like them. They either pay more or, if the transvestite insists upon using the condom, the client will look for another transvestite who does not use one. Clients' rejection of the condom is related to the masculine culture of prison. To use a condom is seen by many men as a precaution associated with the female and the feminine. Moreover, asking prison authorities for a condom involves admitting the person is engaging in homosexual acts, which is both a crime and a stigma. The authorities themselves believe that providing condoms is condoning homosexuality and even confiscate them in routine raids on prisoners' quarters. Under these circumstances, prostitution places the transvestite in an inferior position to his client. His need for money and, as will be seen, his use of drugs makes him particularly vulnerable to his client's demands.

## Alcohol and Drugs

In spite of rigorous prison controls, cocaine, marijuana and barbiturates are easily accessible. Inmates also make '*chicha*', an alcoholic drink made from fermented cereals. The daily consumption of drugs and *chicha* constitutes an important factor in HIV transmission. Another way in which drugs can become a risk of transmission is through the way in which they are distributed. Drugs often enter the prison through visits that women make. The woman hides the drug in a condom in her vagina, and gives it to a transvestite inmate. The transvestite then puts the condom into his rectum. This manoeuvre is done quickly using the same condom, ignoring the risk of HIV transmission implicit in the exchange.

From an analysis of data obtained from openly homosexual men in prison, cocaine use seems also to be related to unprotected anal sex (see Table 6.9). A significant association was also found between alcohol consumption and unprotected receptive anal sex.

## Rape

All of those interviewed reported the danger of rape, which they call *atentados* or 'attempts'. These can occur upon entering the prison or later. On average

*Table 6.9 Prisoners: Unprotected Insertive and Receptive Anal Sex by Type of Drug Consumed*

| | | | Anal penetration without condom | | | | | |
|---|---|---|---|---|---|---|---|---|
| | | | Insertive | | | Receptive | | |
| Drug consumed | Total | | Yes | No | | Yes | No | |
| | (N) | (%) | (N) | (%) | (%) | (N) | (%) | (%) |
| | 22 | 100 | 22 | 32 | 68 | 22 | 68 | 32 |
| Alcohol | | | | | | | | |
| Yes | 18 | 82 | 7 | 86 | 14 | 15 | 93 | 7** |
| No | 4 | 18 | 15 | 80 | 20 | 7 | 57 | 43 |
| Marijuana | | | | | | | | |
| Yes | 19 | 86 | 7 | 86 | 14 | 15 | 93 | 7 |
| No | 3 | 14 | 15 | 86 | 14 | 7 | 71 | 29 |
| Cocaine, acid | | | | | | | | |
| Yes | 13 | 59 | 7 | 86 | 14* | 15 | 73 | 27** |
| No | 9 | 41 | 15 | 47 | 53 | 7 | 29 | 71 |

*The $\chi^2$ of significance indicates a level of significance of 0.10.
**The $\chi^2$ of significance indicates a level of significance of 0.05.

eight inmates were reported as participating in each attempt. The victim is threatened with a sharp weapon, rendering him defenceless to the attack. In these brutal attacks, a condom is not used, creating another source of possible HIV infection. Rape usually occurs during the night in the dormitories and in the lavatories. Victims who resist are injured. When a rape takes place, the victim never reveals the names of the aggressors, because the price may be death. Recovery from this trauma often occurs without the help or knowledge of prison health officials. The motives for such attempts are diverse. On occasion, they occur during the first few days after a transvestite has entered the prison, especially if he does not find a '*padrino*' or godfather to protect him. A transvestite who does not accept sexual propositions from an inmate is also often raped. He may be raped both by the person concerned and by his friends. When a transvestite has entered a gang, obtaining in this way protection in exchange for sex or money, and decides to change gangs, revenge does not wait. Gang rape is the price of desertion.

### Transvestites' Lovers

Most of the one hundred or more transvestites working on the streets of San José live in apartments and houses close to the red light district. Some of them live with their lovers or get together with them in these places. Many of the transvestites' lovers, as opposed to their clients, do not mind being seen with them and are open to be interviewed by people they trust. Given the fact that these lovers make up a group of men who are not perceived as homosexuals, we decided to interview them to find out about their sexual definition, sexual practices, knowledge and beliefs about AIDS and risk of infection.

The first thing that strikes the interviewer is that the gender construction of the men who are the transvestites' lovers is masculine. On searching their past, we found no traces of resistance to rigid roles or to machismo. They are men who for one reason or another have decided to become involved in a relationship with a transvestite. Their lifestyle is similar to any other Costa Rican heterosexual male: married, with children and attracted to feminine qualities. They do not remember, as children, feeling attracted to members of their own sex, or having any feeling of being 'different', as occurs with many men who are gay. Few feel attraction towards men other than transvestites.

Most of the men interviewed are blue-collar workers with very low incomes and little schooling. Juan Carlos sells jelly at a local market and makes about 400 Colones (£2) a day; he used to work as a mechanic and a shoe repairman. Delio is a construction worker who at the present time is not working. Pablo was an accountant for a warehouse but lately he has been out of work and has turned to petty theft. Luis is a hardware store clerk and earns 3,600 Colones per week.

Others are supported by the transvestites such as Moises who says he is with Monique 'for the money'. Pablo lives with what Paula makes, but recognizes that he feels bad about this and states that he used to support her also. Ricardo lives from what Felicia makes and with the money he pays all his expenses. Delio also receives money from Corina because he is unemployed. Not all live off their transvestite partners. David gives 1,000 Colones a week to his transvestite lover. Daniel and Miguel both live with Rita and help her by giving her part of their wages. Jorge does the same with Shasta: they share their salaries to pay the house expenses.

### For Some, Drifting Away from Heterosexuality Is Easy

The history of the men who are transvestites' lovers shows that they have been predominately heterosexual until their relationship with a transvestite. Some, such as José, are married and have children. Miguel had five heterosexual relationships before he met Rita. Daniel has been with transvestites for the past two years but had heterosexual relationships before that. David is 29 and has been in a transvestite relationship for five years; before this, he only had heterosexual encounters and has two children from them.

Despite this past heterosexual activity, they are all very satisfied with their present relationships with transvestites and most, with the exception of Delio and Luis, no longer have any relationships with women. All expressed their preference for a transvestite over a woman, feeling that the transvestite is warmer, more passionate, sexier, and tighter than most women.

### In the Transvestite's World, the Penis Does Not Make the Man

Even though transvestites and their sexual partners are men, this does not mean that their culture is similar to that of the gay community in Costa Rica. In reality, the transvestite and his clients or lovers participate in a sexual culture in which gender takes on a very particular meaning. Transvestites feel like women and are perceived as such, with few exceptions, by their clients and lovers. Being a 'woman' means being 'feminine', and their sexual organs present no obstacle.

For the sexual partner of the transvestite, he is a man and his partner a woman. He expresses his maleness by reporting that he plays only an active or insertive role during anal sex, with very few exceptions. Paula's partner Pablo says that 'he is the man in the relationship'. Melvin says that he is so masculine he does not even want to see the penis of his partner Lina; Luis says the same thing about his partner Salomé, stating that he avoided 'seeing the penis'. In the minds of these men, seeing the transvestite's penis could signify that they were like their clients, or that they are homosexual. On the other hand, Ricardo, who says that he is 'active' in anal sex, states that it does not bother him that his partner has a penis; on the contrary, he likes it because it is different. The only exception was Daniel who admitted that Rita has penetrated him.

The definition of 'man' that a transvestite's lover assumes is no different from that of a heterosexual man. Being a man is to 'screw' a woman or another man. This is why the transvestites' lovers do not feel they are gay or homosexual and for this reason do not participate in gay social activities. Some see themselves as bisexual, others as homosexual, and some as heterosexual, but most see themselves as *cacheros*. Juan Carlos defines a *cachero* as a person who has sex with homosexuals but he himself is not one. Delio defines it as the person who gives pleasure to someone of the same sex. Melvin defines it as a homosexual who acts like a man; Luis interprets it as a man who sleeps with both men and women; David as a 'a man that screws a queer'; and finally, Miguel defines it as a man who makes love to other men.

### Knowledge of AIDS

Transvestites' partners are aware of the danger of AIDS. Juan Carlos knows that AIDS is a threat 'because one is close to the problem', and that the only protection is the use of a condom. Jorge knows that AIDS is transmitted through sexual contact and through blood, and that it has no cure. Moises is just as clear and knows that AIDS is fatal and condoms are the only protection. Although transvestites' lovers know about AIDS, their low income and education has deprived them of the knowledge of preventive medicine. In the National AIDS Survey (Madrigal 1990), it became evident that the groups most opposed to condoms in Costa Rica are precisely those with little education and low income. Additionally, for transvestites' partners, drug dependency complicates the problem.

The fact that most of the transvestites' partners regularly use one or more drugs and that their cost is high (between 1,000 and 12,000 Colones a week) makes them dependent on the transvestites, since their wages would be insufficient to buy them otherwise, especially those who support another household and who have children. Drug use creates additional HIV-related risks, because of the levels of intoxication under which sexual activity is practised and because of depending on others. Lovers depend not only on the transvestite, but also on her sexual customers for their drugs.

### Management of Jealousy

The sexual partners of transvestites define themselves as 'macho' but must consent to being dependent on other men, the transvestites or their clients, in order to satisfy their daily needs. This disempowerment leads them to control and express their jealousy in one of two ways: first, by establishing different rules for jealousy and socialization. In consequence, jealousy is not directed toward clients, but towards other *cacheros*, or other transvestites, thereby breaking ties of solidarity.

The transvestites' lovers have to accept that their partners must prostitute themselves. This makes them feel jealous. Pablo says that 'he feels bad' when Paula is with other men, but he knows why she does it. José is also bothered by Laura sleeping around; 'she does it because she wants to.' Miguel and Daniel who live with Rita are also bothered by prostitution; Miguel recognizes that he is more jealous than the transvestite and Daniel does not like it when Rita prostitutes herself, but 'there is nothing we can do about it'. This case is very special because although they share the same transvestite, although not at the same time, they do not feel jealous towards each other. Moises also believes that when Monique sleeps with others she does it for money, whereas with him she does it for love. Luis is bothered when Salomé sleeps with other men, so he just refuses to visit the place where he knows she works. Salomé says that 'it's the only thing she can do well' and that 'it gives them money for their vices'. Delio recognizes that he is jealous, but not of Corina's prostitution; rather, of her other relationships with other *cacheros*.

The jealousy of the transvestites' lovers is therefore largely directed toward men like themselves. There exists little communication between the *cacheros*. They see themselves as rivals, and friendships between them are rare. This lack of solidarity differentiates the transvestites and their partners from gay men in Costa Rica, who tend to establish closer social relationships.

In the case of AIDS, transvestites' isolation from general society makes them less exposed to information about safer sex and the cultural practices that reinforce it. This is in contrast with gay men who go to bars and follow the norms of the gay community. For transvestites, the practice of safer sex is much more dependent on personal decisions and those of their partners, many of whom do not consider themselves as a group at risk.

A second way of managing jealousy involves establishing different rules about sexual relations for clients and regular partners, including condom use. Most of the transvestites' lovers prefer not to use a condom, even though they are aware that their partners practise prostitution. All feel that the condom diminishes the level of pleasure and view it as something negative. The transvestite views it in a more positive manner but must abide by what the partner wants. This, of course, creates a great obstacle to its use. Laura's partner, José, says he does not use condoms because 'if we are faithful it does not matter, it has been three years and we are still not seropositive'. Even so, he does recognize that it bothers him when Laura gets involved with other men for money. Rita's partner, Miguel, says that he does not like condoms and only uses them every once in a while but he admits he prefers to 'stick it in raw without anything'. Cristina's partner David does not use it either: 'I protect myself, I don't use a condom, I see AIDS like any other venereal disease, like syphilis, gonorrhea, or cancer; one can catch it at any moment. We all have to die some time; a lot of people take care of themselves and they get sick sooner. I don't like to use condoms.'

In view of the fact that these sexual relationships can be potential sources of infection, it is important to discuss the factors that could explain why transvestites' partners do not use condoms. First of all, their low income and educational level place them among those who in Costa Rica most dislike the use of condoms. In the same way, drug and alcohol use puts them at a disadvantage due to intoxication. Another factor is the need to retain power and control. Since the transvestite works as a prostitute, and this is beyond his control, the lover looks to create symbols of his love and affection. He associates prostitution with condom use, and love with unsafe sex. In this way, the lover makes a distinction not only in his sexual role (he is the penetrator), but also in his sexual practice (he does not use a condom).

It is important to appreciate that lovers do love the transvestites. Even though needs and dependencies exist, both hold relationships that are opposed by society and their expressions of love are very evident. Juan Carlos confesses that he loves Monica, and that he does not plan to get married or be with other women because he respects her feelings. Delio plans to continue with Corina because 'she is a beautiful person' even though sometimes other women approach him and he sleeps with them. Melvin loves Lina and he feels hurt that his mother does not accept her. Luis believes that Salomé gives him everything he wants and has introduced her to his brother, who accepts the relationship. Jorge plans to stay with Shasta who 'is superior to all the women he has slept with'.

The fact that many of them are not afraid to go out into the streets with the transvestites, even though they suffer both physical and verbal onslaughts on the street, shows that *cacheros* are willing to take risks. There is more to the relationship than simple curiosity. Many of them admit that it hurts when people make fun of their partners and that has led to fights more than once. A few do not want to be seen with transvestites for fear of losing their job, although they are in the minority. Others who are bolder, like Daniel and Miguel, openly live with their transvestite partner.

It is clear, then, that for both the *cachero* and the transvestite, love is manifested by the actions and risks that each takes to have a relationship. For them, AIDS is just one of many risks that they face. People who love each other do not use condoms and for people who have almost no power, this risk is what little they have to offer as a sign of love. Katia recognizes that 'with her lover she did not use it'. Laura also reports: 'Since my lover did not use it, both of us trusted that we would not harm each other.' Her partner states: 'I don't protect myself when I am with her, because if we are faithful it doesn't matter.' Paula and her partner came to an agreement that she use it with clients but not with him: 'I protect myself against AIDS, I trust Paula in that she uses condoms with other clients since I don't do it with a shirt [condom].'

## Conclusions

It is clear from the evidence cited here that a wide range of behaviourally bisexual men in Costa Rica continue to practise unsafe sex with both male and female partners. Despite having reasonably good knowledge of HIV and AIDS, self-identified bisexual men continue to expose thermselves and their partners to the potential risk of infection, having more unprotected sex with males and females than exclusively homosexual men. Factors militating against the practice of safer sex with women include the perception that vaginal sex is relatively safe, intimacy and trust, and the perceived difficulties of introducing condom use into an on-going relationship.

In prison settings, other factors encourage the continued practice of unsafe sex between men, many of whom are otherwise heterosexual. They include the absence of prison policy on HIV prevention and the non-availability of condoms, guards believing that to distribute condoms is to encourage homosexuality among inmates. Antipathy towards condom use may also be linked to perceptions of masculinity and femininity in prison settings. Taking care of the body and of the self may be seen as unmanly, and to acknowledge the necessity of condom use may be to admit that your prison partner is having sex with other men as well – a symbol of infidelity and an affront to one's prestige and status.

The *cacheros* in the red light district of San José do not wield the power of their counterparts in prison. Their role as protectors is diminished because their transvestite partners must work the streets and are generally the income generators, providing food, shelter and access to drugs. In this kind of situation, lovers' prostitution cannot be denied, and the desire to distinguish between prostitution and love becomes the determining factor over condom use. Here, non-use of the condom becomes a symbol of trust and commitment between lovers, something distinguishing the regular partners of transvestites from clients and the world of the street.

## References

BLUMSTEIN, P. W. and SCHWARTZ, P. (1976a) 'Bisexual Women', in WISEMAN, J. (Ed.), *The Social Psychology of Sex*, New York, Harper & Row.

BLUMSTEIN, P. W. and SCHWARTZ, P. (1976b) 'Bisexuality in Men', *Urban Life*, 5, pp. 339–58.

BODE, J. (1976) *View from Another Closet: Exploring Bisexuality in Women*, New York, Hawthorn Books.

CARRIER, J. M. (1985) 'Mexican Male Bisexuality', in KLEIN, F. and WOLF, T. (Eds) *Two Lives to Lead: Bisexuality in Men and Women*, New York, Harrington Park Press.

CHURCHILL, W. (1967) *Homosexual Behaviour among Males: A Cross-Cultural and Cross-Species Investigation*, New York, Hawthorn Books.

ELLIS, H. (1936) *Studies in the Psychology of Sex*, New York, Mentor Books (originally published 1905).

FISHMAN, J. (1951) *Sex Practices of Prisoners*, New York, Padell Book Co.

FORD, C. S. and BEACH, F. A. (1951) *Patterns of Sexual Behaviour*, New York, Harper (originally published 1934).

HALPERIN, D. M. (1990) *One Hundred Years of Homosexuality and Other Essays on Greek Love*, New York, Routledge.

KINSEY, A. C., POMEROY, W. B. and MARTIN, C. E. (1948) *Sexual Behaviour in the Human Male*, Philadelphia, W.B. Saunders.

KLEIN, F. (1978) *The Bisexual Option*, New York, Arbor House.

KLEIN, F. (1980) 'Are You Sure You Are Heterosexual? Or Homosexual? Or Even Bisexual?', *Forum Magazine*, pp. 41–45.

MACINNES, C. (1973) *Loving Them Both: A Study in Bisexuality and Bisexuals*, London, Dawson.

MADRIGAL, J. (1990) *Primera Encuesta Nacional de SIDA: Informe de Resultados*, San José, Costa Rica, Asociación Demográfica Costaricense.

MONEY, J. (1980) *Love and Love Sickness*, Baltimore, Johns Hopkins University Press.

SCOTT, J. C. (pseud.) (1978) *Wives who Love Women*, New York, Walker.

SCHIFTER, J. and MADRIGAL, J. (1992) *Hombres que Aman Hombres*, San José, Costa Rica, ILEP-SIDA.

TVERSKY, A. and KAHNEMAN, D. (1973) 'Availability: A Heuristic for Judging Frequency and Probability', *Cognitive Psychology*, 4, pp. 207–32.

WARREN, C. A. B. (1974) *Identity and Community in the Gay World*, New York, John Wiley and Sons.

*Chapter 7*

# AIDS and the Enigma of Bisexuality in the Dominican Republic

*E. Antonio de Moya and Rafael García*

So there is no comparison between the two things; one person likes one, another likes the other; I like both. (*Anthologia Palatina*, I.65, trans. W. R. Patton, quoted in Boswell, 1981, p. 74)

There are indeed many precautions to imprison a man into what he is, as if we lived in perpetual fear that he might escape from it, that he might break away and suddenly elude this condition. (J. P. Sartre, *Being and Nothingness*, 1943)

Bi-eroticism, bisexual behaviour, and bisexuality have frequently been described as elusive concepts and highly misunderstood phenomena (Tannahill, 1980; Klein and Wolf, 1985) which have defied scientific explanation since the ancient times of Greek tolerant views of bisexual pederasty (Travin and Protter, 1993). Twentieth-century theorists from Freud (1905) onwards, have speculated that bisexuality is a fundamental human characteristic, and that socialization is responsible for the development of either hetero- or homoeroticism. However, bi-eroticism and bisexuality have not been extensively studied, and the mechanisms whereby sexual orientation is shaped have yet to be explicated (Bancroft, 1989; Levine, 1992). Most conceptual models of bisexuality explain it in terms of conflictual or confused identity development, retarded sexual development, or a defence against 'true' heterosexuality or homosexuality. It has been suggested, however, that some individuals can eroticize more than one love object regardless of gender (Hansen, 1985), that sexual patterns could be more variable and fluid than theoretical notions tend to allow, and that sexual desire may not be as fixed and static in individuals as is assumed by 'essential' sexual categories and identities (Paul, 1985).

It has also been proposed that in the psychosocial sphere, the differentiation of the sexes proceeds from an original state of bisexuality (Abraham, 1948). Kinsey *et al.* (1948) found that about three-quarters of American men who were not exclusively heterosexual reported behaving bisexually. Money (1968) argued that homosexual activity at the time of puberty and early adolescence is more prevalent than is generally conceded. Weinberg (1976) asserts that bisexuals are more likely to associate with heterosexuals and are more concerned to pass as non-homosexuals. Gagnon (1977) points out that the question to be asked is what kind of learning histories and contexts make sex with both genders possible, while Zinick (1985) states that a bisexual self-identity can be maintained over time, in which dual sexual interests and behaviour are successfully integrated into an overall lifestyle.

The advent of HIV and AIDS has brought renewed interest in bisexual behaviour and bisexuality because of the presumption that bisexual men are responsible for 'transferring' HIV infection from the male homosexual population to the heterosexual population, and vice versa. Guimaraes, Terto and Parker (1992), Parker (1993) and Guimaraes (1994) found that many HIV positive Brazilian women unknowingly had bisexual partners who were HIV infected and who practised anal sex. Generally in Latin America, if a male partner assumes the insertive role during homosexual relations, his male gender identity may not be threatened, as only the receptive male is considered to be homosexual (Akers, 1973; Carrier, 1985). In the Dominican Republic, where 70 per cent of the AIDS cases reported between 1983 and 1986 were among homosexual and bisexual men, the epidemic soon became predominantly heterosexual, with a male to female ratio of 2:1 in the general population (Garris *et al.*, 1991), and a ratio of 1:1 among HIV positive Haitian and Dominican–Haitian sugar-cane plantation workers and their wives (Capellán, 1992). But little is known about the possible influence of male bisexual behaviour in bringing about this change. Two parallel epidemics, one predominantly homosexual, and the other heterosexual, may have started simultaneously, or bisexual males may have served as an epidemic 'bridge' for the transmission of HIV infection from homosexual males to heterosexual women. A closer look at historical roots of bisexual behaviour in this country, the variety of its present sociocultural manifestations, and recent research findings related to risk of HIV infection in bisexual men and their heterosexual and homosexual partners is badly needed, as HIV prevention should take into account both the persistence of, and the meanings attached by social groups to different ways of sexual interaction.

### The Historical Roots

Although same-sex practices between men in the Americas date back to pre-colonial times (Freyre, 1946), little is known about the sexual culture of South American Arawak polysynthetic societies, and their Caribbean descendants prior to the arrival of Europeans. As early as 1535, Gonzalo Fernández de Oviedo, one of the first colonial governors of La Hispaniola island, shared today by Haiti and the Dominican Republic, wrote about male and female bisexuality as well as homosexuality, anal intercourse, women's anxiety about homosexual relations between men, and the *berdache* ('half man–half woman') tradition (Oviedo/Las Casas, 1988):

Cacique (chief) Behechio had thirty wives, not only for the kind of intercourse which married men are naturally used to have with them, but for other beastly and unspeakable sins. . . . Cacique Goacanagarix had certain women with whom he had intercourse in the way vipers have. . . . But if there is such a fame about this cacique, it is clear that he would not be the only one doing such unspeakable and dirty crime; for common people (and even the whole reign) then procure to imitate their prince in their virtues and vices. . . . What I have said of these people is very public on this and neighbouring islands, and even in the continent, where *many of these male and female Indians were sodomites*. . . . Indeed, this is a very usual, ordinary and common thing among them. . . . And you should know that the man who plays patient or takes the position of being the woman in that beastly and anathematized act is given the role of a woman, and wears *naguas* (skirts) as women do. . . . This abominable *contra natura* sin was very usual among the male Indians of this island; but to women it was abhorrent, because of their own interest rather than because of any scruples of consciousness. . . . (pp. 146–8, translation ours; emphasis added)

The historian John Boswell (1981) argues that European theological discussions of the Middle Ages resulted in the establishment of rigid standards of faith to which Christians must adhere or face the power of the Inquisition. Compared to colonizers' attitudes toward sex, native North Americans, for example, seemed to be more uninhibited, and were innocent of the notion that something they enjoyed might be 'wrong' (Blevins, 1973). From Fernández de Oviedo's account, it seems evident that the dominant Christian sex-conflict paradigm and the subordinate Caribbean sex-flexible paradigm immediately clashed. The social and political result of this conflict was the virtual genocide of the aboriginal population within a few decades, and the utilitarian conversion to Christianity of indigenous survivors and their descendants. Dominican historians have traditionally assumed that the aborigine culture soon became extinguished because of the hardships of the conquering process. A reinterpretation of this notion argues that extensive miscegenation practices between male Spanish settlers and native women taken as concubines allowed for the subsumption, reverse colonization, clandestinization, and survival of indigenous cultural patterns under the guise of dominant colonial culture, through the primary socialization of the new *mestizo* or *criollo* (creole) children by indigenous mothers (De Moya, 1993).

Sexual practices newly defined as 'transgressive' (Parker, 1991) seemed to survive as an underground culture among American–European descendants. The new official mediaeval Catholic standards became the yardsticks against which social behaviour would be measured. *Mestizos* identifying with the dominant class should be publicly over-compliant with formal Christian marriage rules, although privately they retained polygamous practices through serial concubinage. They also displayed a strong public homophobia, although comradeship and enduring friendship between males continued to be perceived as superior to relationships with females, who were frequently seen as 'cunning' and 'treacherous,' the only exception being one's own mother, who was regarded as a saint. From those days on, it seems that inhabitants of the island utilized a paradoxical logic through which the simultaneous denial and assertion of the self became a generalized approach to social life, a magical resolution of Hamlet's dilemma ('to be' *or* 'not to be'), in which 'to be' *and* 'not to be' could smoothly coalesce and be confounded with each other.

To complicate things further, a new breed of enslaved people from various African territories were imported into the island early in the sixteenth century. Surviving native females interbred with runaway African males, giving rise to the *cimarrones* (bush-people), the forerunners of today's Dominican lower and lower-middle classes, who publicly endorse a compound matrist-patrist religious approach,[1] and a more flexible outlook on gender roles and sexual behaviour. On the other hand, *mestizo* and subordinate Spanish males interbred extensively with enslaved African females, giving rise in the main part to today's middle and upper-middle classes, who publicly endorse a patrist Catholic religious stance, and display more restrictive bipolar gender roles and sexual behaviours. It is hardly surprising that all this interaction and blending of American, European and African ethnic groups and cultures in a small island should create a peculiar society.

An interesting example of colonial social treatment of powerful European males' bisexual behaviour in this island is offered by anthropologist Carlos E. Deive (1988):

> Juan de Echegoian, a Spanish judge who lived in La Hispaniola from 1547 to 1564, married to doña Andrea, made a sexual proposal to 16-year-old Hernando de Bascones, from Seville, and to Antonio Jácome, a Portuguese youth. . . . The latter denounced the judge to the Royal Audience on the grounds that he had tempted both him and Bascones to commit the 'unspeakable crime'. . . . Echegoian was subject to ridicule and public scorn . . . although his skills as a lawyer enabled him to escape prosecution for this and other accusations, such as anally sodomizing a female slave concubine. (pp. 101–2, translation ours)

About a hundred years later, in 1664, the first publicized episode of mass harassment against men of *ambigui generis*, known in those days as *mariones*, occurred. Many of these men were likely to be behaviourally bisexual, because of the general imposition of heterosexual marriage on adult men. According to Deive (1988):

It all started when Juan Pérez, a soldier and barber of the municipal penitentiary, made a sexual proposal to a Spanish settler, who denounced him to the Audience. . . . Under torture, Pérez confessed not only his attraction to men, but also that of others. Colonial President Pedro Carvajal y Cobos himself headed the investigation during several nights, which led to many arrests. More accusations arose from enquiries of defendants, and from these others, and as a chain reaction, there were tortures, confessions and sentences. . . . Six of the culprits were sentenced to be burned, but only in four of them was this done, as the two others successfully appealed. A minor of age was passed through the flames, received a hundred lashes of the whip and was banished from the island. Another was mutilated and the rest suffered the same punishment as the minor. Satisfied, President Carvajal y Cobos reported to the king about the extinction 'of that spark'. (pp. 103–4, translation ours)

As centuries went by, tacit tolerance of widespread heterosexual concubinage and extra-marital relationships, and a reluctant acceptance of occasional homosexual and bisexual relationships, along with official attempts at repression and suppression of these practices when political convenience dictated it, dominated the social scenario. In the twentieth century, during Rafael Trujillo's dictatorship (1930–61), homophobic authoritarianism seemed to reach its peak. A homosexual or bisexual orientation or identity was regarded as a family disgrace and shame, which could retroactively implicate family members and ancestors as 'carriers' of this weakness of character. Homosexual and bisexual males were frequently subject to blackmail and aggression, ostracized, or even driven to commit suicide. Many were also forced by social pressure to marry women and to father children, as a means of disavowing the imputation of homosexuality. In the early 1950s, Trujillo went so far as to create two concentration camps for middle- and upper-middle-class intellectual and/or political male dissidents suspected of being, or known to be, homosexual or bisexual, but this control measure was short-lived because of strong societal resistance.

The fashionable Latin American machismo of those days represented the homosexual man, mostly those known to be the orally or anally receptive partner in sexual intercourse, as someone who sooner or later would show the symptoms of feminine degeneracy, and who could transmit these properties to other males socially interacting with him. Bisexual men were called *redondos* (round men), and were often seen as deceptive or covert homosexuals. Young boys with androgynous or feminine attributes were a source of embarrassment to parents and other close relatives, and were stringently socialized in 'men's things', such as forcibly having sexual intercourse with female sex workers at an early age (García and Renshaw, 1987; García *et al.*, 1994).

### The Construction of Masculinity

At the onset of puberty, the Dominican boy, mostly in the less restrictive matrifocal lower socio-economic classes, seems to develop a secret but uninhibited polymorphous sexual orientation, which may include copulation into hand-made 'vaginal' orifices of porous trees, individual and group secret zoophilic experiences, group masturbation contests, as well as clandestine and 'innocent' love affairs with cousins and peers, with no awareness or self-attribution of homosexuality. Scientific knowledge on the present prevalence of bisexual behaviour from puberty onwards in the Dominican society is scarce, although anecdotal evidence suggests that it may be extensively practised in secret by males. If this is true at least among young male adolescents, and between older male adolescents and adults, it is necessary to study the cultural norms that facilitate its occurrence. It is not clear how many of the men who exhibit bisexual behaviour during adolescence continue to do so in adulthood, and how many end up identifying themselves as heterosexual, homosexual, or bisexual. Because of their stigmatized, clandestine and self-denying nature, these transactions could pose a real risk of HIV transmission to both the male and female populations, particularly to adolescents and youths.

Many men's apparent attraction to sexual partners of both sexes, and their presumed interest in sexually 'subordinating' or being 'subordinated' by other men via oral and/or anal penetration, appears to be socially understood as a test of their degree of masculinity. This tradition seems to stem from mixed Mediterranean and African conceptions of male sexuality linked both to ideas of phallicism (and its attendant phallocracy) and to homophobia, an irrational fear of the male acquisition of female properties by being anally receptive. The merging of these two notions have resulted in a *machista* construction of masculinity which appears to be centered around the use a male makes of his anus rather than on the use he makes of his genitals, as only the male who is anally receptive by choice 'loses' his masculine attributes.

It is not clear at what point in history femininity and receptiveness came to be regarded as synonymous categories, but Boswell (1981) points out that a strong bias already existed against receptive sexual behaviour on the part of adult male citizens in ancient Rome, although foreigners, slaves, and youths could engage in such behaviour without loss of status. But if an adult citizen openly indulged in such behaviour, he was viewed with scorn. The most common distinction was between insertive (*exoleti*) and receptive (*catamiti*) male sex workers. Male brothels employed men with large penises, and large genital endowment among males elicited much comment among Roman writers.

Boswell (1981) also mentions the French word *bougre* ('bugger' in English), commonly used for heretics of Bulgarian origin, a term which came to refer to a person who practised 'sodomy'. By the sixteenth century, the term 'buggery' was used in English law to designate homosexuality. Nowadays, this word is translated in the Dominican Republic as *bugarrón* to designate the anal inserter, usually a sex worker, the antonym of *maricón*, which designates the anal receptor.

### The Joint Operation of Phallicism and Homophobia

In Dominican society, the cult to the large and wide *sacred phallus*, vested with magical-religious, erotic, and political powers, is a driving force in the socialization of boys, as well as a social temptation for the initiation of male-to-male competitive sexual relations which validate gender-role definitions through transgression. Across the island, short penis size in a newborn is seen as a hindrance, while a large penis is usually associated with community curiosity, fascination, praise, and likely success in future love affairs. In Haiti, for example, a small stone is hung by a thin cord to the short penis of boys in order to enlarge their genitals (Del Cabral, 1987), and in the Dominican Republic young men socially compete with each other over genital endowment, conferring special privileges upon the winner, which might include, in some instances, orally or anally penetrating peers in secret encounters. The penis size of boys is usually known to relatives, and proudly communicated to neighbours and friends. Having a large penis is seen as lowering resistance to sexual temptation and with early sexual initiation with an older female or male via seduction. Usually, the younger, weaker, and less experienced the boy is, the more likely he is to end up as the receptive partner in homosexual intercourse. Small groups of boys, mostly in the lower socio-economic classes, often conduct *maniguas* (gang rape) to initiate their newest members. These establish a power hierarchy among them. Another relatively common practice among older adolescents and young adults is *misas negras* ('Black Sabbaths' or orgies), in which an uneven number of shifting partners of both sexes participate, forcing the formation of successive bisexual triangles. More enduring and affectionate secret 'husband-wife' relationships between boys and male adolescents are also known to occur, as is the 'renting' of receptive boys to homosexual or bisexual adults by the boys' peers.

Parents strongly fear that their children could become homosexual and, because of this, the mother tends to become the guardian of their sexuality, probably in order to avoid casting aspersions on the father's masculinity. A series of important research questions derive from these observations. Is it true that Dominican women have a stronger aversion to male homosexual behaviour than heterosexual males, because of fear of losing male partners due to other males' competition, as Oviedo (1535) seems to suggest? Is a conflicting approach-avoidance phallicist *and* homophobic attitude induced by parents in young boys by emphasizing strict gender-role differences which may generalize to same-sex social interaction? What mechanisms do families adopt to prevent or control 'transgressive' cross-gender behaviour in males suspected of being 'different' during childhood, puberty, and adolescence? Is a 'receptive' homosexual identity regarded as an individual disadvantage and a family shame because of beliefs in the inferiority of women?

Paradoxically, under special borderline circumstances such as being the only boy in a family of sisters, or being the last boy in a long family, feminine behaviour in boys with androgynous characteristics may be tolerated and reinforced by mothers in order to ensure boys' allegiance in old age, but most often by grandmothers to whom these children are often given for companionship and exemplary socialization. In these rearing practices, many of the characteristics of the *berdache* seem to survive nowadays.[2]

Modern *berdaches* in the Dominican society take the form of urban *travestis* (transvestites), sugar-cane plantation *masissís* (boy-girls or men-women), and to a lesser extent, small-town *señoritos* ('mama's boys'). *Travestis* usually work either as socially 'heterosexual' female street sex workers in large cities, or as highly popular female impersonators in nightclubs all around the country. *Masissís* are Haitian or Dominican–Haitian males usually born with a *sacred phallus*, who are reared by their families as social females, regarded by the community as 'very expensive women', and who may be prospective *houngans* (vodu priests) because of their genital 'blessing'. The *señorito* is usually socialized as an overprotected house boy, often dressed in white clothes, and never put on the floor to avoid becoming dirty. He is supposed to be devoted to his family, a likely Church acolyte during puberty, chaste in his adolescence, heterosexually monogamous and faithful to his only wife, and a good father to his children. Although most *señoritos* spend their adolescence under close surveillance by their caretakers, they tend to become the community's *forbidden fruits* for both males and females, and as such are highly vulnerable to seduction, a reason why some of them end up involved in relatively stable sexual relationships with either bisexual or homosexual men. Many of these modern *berdaches* are not exclusively receptive homosexuals as might be expected, but transgress the rules by playing the insertive role with homosexual, bisexual, and even 'curious' heterosexual men, as well as women, mostly because of their readiness to provide satisfaction in either or both ways to sexual partners.

## Clandestine Bisexual Arrangements

Relationships among young men have an unconscious, ambivalent, and erotic overtone and are generally approved by one or both friends' families, provided that neither of the friends is suspected of being 'effeminate' and both show a proper erotic interest in girls or women in their daily talk. In many cases, 'passing' strategies are developed in order to maintain the secrecy of these bonds, in situations where male partners may not even know that what they do with each other is understood as homosexual behaviour, and both may sequentially or simultaneously have non-suspecting girlfriends. Some of the most successful passing strategies include self-presentation as '*hermanos del alma'* (soul brothers), *hermanos de sangre* (blood brothers), *primos hermanos* (first cousins), or *inseparables como uña y dedo* ('inseparable as nail and finger'). Another common passing strategy entails establishing highly respectable family bonds, such as becoming *cuñados* (brothers-in-law), i.e. becoming the boyfriend or husband one's of male lover's sister, or becoming *compadres* (the godfather) of the male lover's newborn child. These hidden homosexual relations complement heterosexual relations, and usually pass unnoticed by non-suspecting girlfriends or wives.

### Bisexuality among Homotropic Sex Workers

Because of the homophobic phallicist tradition, many young men in the Dominican Republic sell sex to other men while participating in heterosexual sex for pleasure. Frías and Lara (1987), for example, found that 28 per cent of lower-class, 18 per cent of middle-class, and 8 per cent of upper-class 17- to 28-year-old males in Santo Domingo had practised some kind of homosexual behaviour in their lifetime, two-thirds of them also having intercourse with women. By the age of 14 or 15, lower-class boys in particular learn that, in adult sexual culture, sex has a price and might produce money; that there is a cult to virginity and youth; and that there is a relatively constant adult demand for casual and anonymous sex (De Moya, 1987). This culture paves the way for engaging in bisexual behaviour without having to self-identify as homosexual. Recent anthropological and epidemiological studies in the Dominican Republic have identified at least three lower-class groups which exhibit such behaviour in association with paid sex, namely *palomos* (behaviourally bisexual homeless boys), *bugarrones* (bisexual 'homotropic' sex workers), and *Sanky-Pankies* (bisexually oriented sex workers), who are reminiscent of Roman *exoleti* prostitutes, but who might also transgress the rules vis-à-vis a more masculine partner and behave as *catamiti*.

### Bisexual Behaviour and Risk of HIV

In an early qualitative study, De Moya (1987) found that *palomos* start having sex at about the age of 10–11. By 14–15, male peers start putting pressure on these prospective *bugarrones* to go with *maricones* in order to demonstrate that they are not *pendejos* ('jerks' or 'chicken'), as they should show an interest in money and not be afraid of men. The financial gain linked to the transaction tends to satisfy both basic needs and to strip homosexual behaviour of its stigma, offering the *bugarrón* an alibi for sexually relating to men while denying any personal involvement or interest in this behaviour. Homeless young men who sell sex have to exhibit a pose of emotional detachment from their clients, sharing with peers the financial gains, and spending money on girlfriends and female sex workers in order to avoid being discredited and losing status in the group. Publicly, they must emphasize that they only like women, and when possible, they must 'pimp' for one or more female sex workers as a demonstration of manliness.

Such boys know little about sexually transmitted diseases and HIV infection. Transmission is attributed mostly to bad luck, with high levels of irrelevant antibiotic self-medication, and the use of home-made herbal preparations. The existence of an HIV asymptomatic state is understood, but they do not believe that any of their clients could have been infected. Condom use is not perceived as necessary if the client is a known, clean, and trusted person. There is also a tendency for clients to prefer younger virgin boys, as these are perceived as having a lower risk of being HIV infected.

Ruíz and Vásquez (1993) conducted a quantitative study with a sample of seventy-six lower-class sex workers/*bugarrones* in Santo Domingo. Thirty-nine per cent were aged 13–17, 49 per cent were 18–24, and 12 per cent were older than 24, mostly acting as *maipiolos* (matchmakers) for younger ones. One-third were illiterate, homeless, or already had children. All had had vaginal intercourse and 41 per cent had had anal intercourse with women, initiating these practices by the age of 13. They had a median of twenty-four different female partners per year, 43 per cent had had intercourse with female sex workers, and 26 per cent defined themselves as *chulos* or pimps. In their last five insertive heterosexual relations, only 19 per cent said they had consistently used condoms, 40 per cent had used them inconsistently, and 41 per cent had not used them at all.

Homosexual relations were initiated between 14 and 15 years of age, in 65 per cent of cases because of economic need. The mean number of male clients was thirty-six per year. The mean number of foreign tourist male clients was seventeen during lifetime, a relationship they prefer because it is better paid and usually less sexually threatening, with a lower demand for receptive anal sex. Receptive anal and/or oral sex for pleasure was seen as a highly stigmatizing practice by nine out of ten respondents, but about one-third did not regard these practices as an identifying criterion, provided they got enough cash or valuable gifts from clients. Insertive anal sex with men had been practised by 90 per cent of respondents, 39 per cent of whom said they always used condoms. Nearly one-third admitted they had practised receptive oral and/or anal sex for money, 33 per cent had practised oral sex for pleasure, and 12 per cent had practised receptive anal sex for pleasure. Fear of dying was a motive for AIDS prevention for 68 per cent of participants, followed by fear of not being able to procreate healthy children (58 per cent), fear of not being able to help support their mothers (55 per cent), fear of losing their physical attractiveness (47 per cent), and fear of having to abandon sexual activity (42 per cent).

In a broader context, Ramah et al. (1992) conducted interviews with 188 men who had sex with men between the ages of 14 and 47, in five Dominican cities. Nearly two-thirds of respondents had also had sex with women at some time in their lives. Those who had had this experience also tended to be the

insertive partners in their male-to-male behaviour, represented a disproportionate percentage of those who have had a sexually transmitted disease, and
were more likely to have received payment for sex. Forty-five per cent of the
whole sample classified themselves as homosexual, 38 per cent as bisexual,
and 17 per cent as heterosexual. Only 38 per cent had consistently used
condoms in their last five encounters with men. Among respondents who
stated they had had sex with men for money, 64 per cent also reported having
sex with women. Sixty-six per cent of those who had had sex with women
reported not using condoms during vaginal or anal sex in the last twelve
months. Behaviourally bisexual men tended to have a lower socio-economic
status, presently have a female sexual partner, and identify themselves as
having insertive sex for money mostly with older receptive upper-middle class
and foreign male tourists.

Silvestre *et al.* (1994) studied 412 children aged 12–17 years, involved in
sex work in five Dominican cities. They estimate that around 25,000 children
in the country presently sell sex, with a ratio of two girls for every boy. Girls
tend to work in bars and brothels, catering to a male clientele, whereas boys
tended to work on the streets, in parks, and on beaches, catering to both male
and female clients. Boys' involvement in sex work was attributed mostly to
poverty. The age of initiation into sex work for boys was 11–12 years, with a
tendency to decrease in younger recruits. Younger boys (12–15 years old)
tended to attract the oldest male clients. In beach towns, from 65 to 88 per
cent of boys' clients were foreign tourists; only one-third of boys used condoms with men.

Male bisexuals' sex work with foreign tourists was studied by De Moya *et
al.* (1992) with twenty-two males known as *Sanky-Pankies* ('Hanky-Pankies' or
'beach boys') in Sosúa, a small town on the northern coast of the country. As
a result of the development of tourism, gigolism (i.e. living off foreign visitors
of either sex) has developed. Institutionalized in the late 1970s and 1980s,
such practices have been reinforced by the xenophilic attitudes among many
Dominicans, who perceive tourists as rich people who might help them escape
poverty through migration to more developed countries.

The median age of respondents was 22 years. Their average schooling was
fifth grade. Five were married and seventeen were single. They estimated that
half of the *Sankies* used to sexually relate to male tourists in the 1980s, but
nowadays the number has decreased to two of every ten, because of
homophobia reinforced by fear of AIDS. Only one participant said that 'many'
of them still have intercourse with men. Nevertheless, a 12-year-old 'gigolo'
apprentice (*secretario*) was asked whether the boy could introduce him to a
bisexual *Sanky*. The boy just pointed to one of the interviewees, who ran away
from him in an apparent display of embarrassment. Four participants had
known at least one bisexual *Sanky* who had died of AIDS or had the disease.
Not having vaginal intercourse with women was a rare event for them. They
reported a median of twenty lifetime female tourist partners. Only one stated
that he had practised anal sex with women. Five admitted they never offered

condom protection to women, and nine asserted they always used condoms. Reasons why they did not use condoms included drunkenness, desperation, feeling the sensation of skin contact, trust, and love.

## Conclusions

Bi-eroticism, bisexual behaviour, and bisexuality seem to be inherent in the social construction of masculinity and gender-role relationships among many Dominican males. A strong stigma is still, however, attached to the publicly known receptive partner in male homosexual intercourse, as a consequence of beliefs in the masculinity/femininity power distinction. In the process of developing a sexual identity, many young men exhibit an approach-avoidance conflict which confounds affiliation, competition, and domination towards members of their own sex. A complex matrix of phallicist, homophobic, pederastic, and xenophilic attitudes, characteristic of today's Dominican culture, both attracts and repels young men from each other. This conflict, probably reinforced by a fear of women's likely homophobic attitudes and behaviour, tends to sustain among bisexual males a high level of impulsive clandestine behaviour, deceptiveness to female partners, and infidelity to male partners, with short-lived affective bonds, guilt and self-denial.

The notion that bisexual men's behaviour may serve as a likely 'bridge' for the transmission of sexually transmitted diseases and HIV is reinforced by research which indicates that no less than two in every three males who have sex with males also have sex with females. Extensive and frequent unprotected receptive anal sex for money, practised at least by one-third of these men, mostly lower-class youths, increases their risk of acquiring HIV infection and of transmitting it to other unsuspecting male and female partners. Gender-role flexibility with no condom protection during sexual intercourse constitutes a special case for immediate action by the National AIDS Program, and these males and their partners should be actively included in HIV prevention initiatives culturally sensitive to their little-understood behaviour.

## Notes

1  *Santería* and *vodu* are syncretic Caribbean cults in which African and indigenous deities 'pass' as Catholic saints.
2  *Berdache* is a term derived from a Persian word meaning 'kept boy' or 'male prostitute', applied by French explorers to designate the receptive partners in homosexual relationships between native American males (Trimmer, 1978). The *berdache* has been defined as a person of one sex, who assumed the gender role of the other sex, cross-dressing as part of the assumed role (Midnight Sun, 1988). He/she was often the tribe or band's medicine-person, doctor, story teller, matchmaker, or leading scalp dancer. Certain

taboos in particular tribes forbade their high priest to marry women and father children. Women were rarely taken on war parties because, should a woman begin to menstruate, her blood might bring defeat (Kenny, 1988).

## References

ABRAHAM, K. (1948) *Selected Papers of Karl Abraham*, The International Psycho-analytic Library, London, The Hogarth Press.

AKERS, R. L. (1973) *Deviant Behaviour: A Social Learning Approach*, Belmont, California, Wadsworth Publishing Co.

BANCROFT, J. (1989) *Human Sexuality and its Problems*, London, Churchill Livingstone.

BLEVINS, W. (1973) *Give Your Hearts to the Hawks: A Tribute to the Mountain Men*, Los Angeles, Nash Publishing.

BOSWELL, J. (1981) *Christianity, Social Tolerance, and Homosexuality*, Chicago, University of Chicago Press.

CAPELLÁN, M. (1992) *Prevalencia de Infecciones por VIH y HTLV-1 en Bateyes Dominicanos*, MD Thesis, Universidad Autónoma de Santo Domingo.

CARRIER, J. M. (1985) 'Mexican Male Bisexuality', in KLEIN, F. and WOLF, T. (Eds) *Two Lives to Lead: Bisexuality in Men and Women*, New York, Harrington Park Press.

DEIVE, C. E. (1988) *La Mala Vida. Delincuencia y Picaresca en la Colonia Española de Santo Domingo*, Santo Domingo, Fundación Cultural Dominicana.

DEL CABRAL, M. (1987) *El Escupido*, Santo Domingo, Editora De Colores.

DE MOYA, E. A. (1987) *La Alfombra de Guazabara o el Reino de los Desterrados*, paper presented at the First Dominican Congress on Homeless Children, Santo Domingo.

DE MOYA, E. A. (1993) 'Animación sociocultural y polisíntesis en la transformación del sistema educativo dominicano', *Revista del Plan Decenal de Educación*, 1, 1.

DE MOYA, E. A., GARCÍA, R., FADUL, R. and HEROLD, E. (1992) 'Sosua's Sanky-Pankies and Female Sex Workers', unpublished manuscript, Instituto de Sexualidad Humana, Universidad Autónoma de Santo Domingo.

FREUD, S. (1961) 'Three Essays on the Theory of Sexuality', in STRACHEY, J. (Ed. and Trans.) *The Standard Edition of the Complete Psychological Works of Sigmund Freud* (Vol. 7), London, The Hogarth Press (original work published 1905).

FREYRE, G. (1946) *The Masters and the Slaves*, New York, Alfred Knopf.

FRÍAS, M. M. and LARA, S. S. (1987) *Actitudes y comportamiento sexual en hombres de 18–27 años en Santo Domingo*, BA thesis, Psychology Department, Universidad Autónoma de Santo Domingo.

GAGNON, J. (1977) *Human Sexualities*, Glenview, IL, Scott Foresman.

GARCÍA, R. and RENSHAW, D. (1987) 'A Contemporary Prostitution Accepting Culture', *British Journal of Sexual Medicine*, 14, 3, pp. 72–5.

GARCÍA, R., FADUL, R., DE MOYA, E. A., GÓMEZ, E. and HEROLD, E. (1992) *Conducta Sexual del Adolescente Dominicano*, Santo Domingo, Instituto de Sexualidad Humana, Universidad Autónoma de Santo Domingo.

GARCÍA, R., DE MOYA, E. A., FADUL, R., FREITES, A., GUERRERO, S. and CASTELLANOS, C. (1994) 'Counselors' and HIV-Positive Patients' Perceptions of Gender Differences in HIV/AIDS Education and Counseling', in WIJEYARATNE, P., ROBERTS, J. H., KITTS, L. and ARSENAULT, L. J. (Eds) *Gender, Health, and Sustainable Development: A Latin American Perspective*, Ottawa, International Development Research Centre.

GARRIS, I., RODRÍGUEZ, E., DE MOYA, E. A., MONTERROSSO, E., GUERRERO, E. and GÓMEZ, E. (1991) 'AIDS Heterosexual Predominance in the Dominican Republic', *Journal of Acquired Immune Deficiency Syndrome*, 4, pp. 1173–8.

GUIMARAES, C. D. (1994) 'Male Bisexuality, Gender Relations, and AIDS in Brazil', in WIJEYARATNE, P., ROBERTS, J. H., KITTS L. and ARSENAULT, L. J. (Eds) *Gender, Health, and Sustainable Development: A Latin American Perspective*, Ottawa, International Development Research Centre.

GUIMARAES, C. D., TERTO, V. and PARKER, R. G. (1992) 'Homossexualidade, bissexualidade HIV/AIDS no Brasil: Uma bibliografia anotada das Ciencias Sociais', *Physis: Jornal de Saúde Coletiva*, 2, 1, 151–83.

HANSEN, C. E. (1985) 'Bisexuality Reconsidered: An Idea in Pursuit of a Definition', in KLEIN, F. and WOLF, T. (Eds) *Two Lives to Lead: Bisexuality in Men and Women*, New York, Harrington Park Press.

KENNY, M. (1988) 'Tinseled Bucks: A Historical Study in Indian Homosexuality', in ROSCOE, W. (Ed.) *Living the Spirit*, New York, St Martin's Press.

KINSEY, A., POMEROY, C. and MARTIN, C. E. (1948) *Sexual Behaviour in the Human Male*, New York, W.B. Saunders.

KLEIN, F. and WOLF, T. (Eds) (1985) *Two Lives to Lead: Bisexuality in Men and Women*, New York, Harrington Park Press.

LEVINE, S. B. (1992) *Sexual Life: A Clinician's Guide*, New York, Plenum Press.

MIDNIGHT SUN (1988) 'Sex/Gender Roles in Native North America', in ROSCOE, W. (Ed.) *Living the Spirit*, New York, St Martin's Press.

MONEY, J. (1968) *Gay, Straight, and In-Between*, New York, Oxford University Press.

OVIEDO/LAS CASAS (1988) *Crónicas Escogidas*, Santo Domingo, Ediciones de la Fundación Corripio.

PARKER, R. G. (1991) *Bodies, Pleasures, and Passions. Sexual Culture in Contemporary Brazil*, Boston, Beacon Press.

PARKER, R. G. (1993) 'Sexo entre Homens: Consciencia da AIDS e comportamento sexual entre os homens homossexuais e bissexuais no Brasil', in PARKER, R. G. *et al.* (Eds) *AIDS no Brasil*, Relume Dumará, ABIA, IMS-Uerj.

PAUL, J. P. (1985) 'Bisexuality: Reassessing Our Paradigms of Sexuality', in KLEIN, F. and WOLF, T. (Eds) *Two Lives to Lead: Bisexuality in Men and Women*, New York, Harrington Park Press.

RAMAH, M., PAREJA, R. and HASBÚN, J. (1992) 'Dominican Republic: Lifestyles and Sexual Practices. Results of KABP Conducted among Homosexual and Bisexual Men', unpublished manuscript, Santo Domingo, USAID/AIDSCAP.

RECHY, J. (1959) 'The Fabulous Wedding of Miss Destiny', *BigTable*, 1, 3.

RECHY, J. (1961) 'A Quarter Ahead', *Evergreen Review*, 5, 19, p. 18.

REISS, A. (1964) 'The Social Integration of Queers and Peers', in BECKER, H. S. (Ed.) *The Other Side: Perspectives on Deviance*, New York, Free Press.

ROSS, H. L. (1959) 'The "Hustler" in Chicago', *The Journal of Student Research*, 1, pp. 13–19.

RUÍZ, C. and VÁSQUEZ, R. E. (1993) *Características psicosociales y motivación para la prevención del SIDA en trabajadores sexuales homotrópicos*, BA thesis, Department of Psychology, Universidad Autónoma de Santo Domingo.

SARTRE, J. P. (1943) *Being and Nothingness*, Paris, Gallimarol.

SILVESTRE, E., RIJO, J. and BOGAERT, H. (1994) *La neo-prostitución infantil en República Dominicana*, Santo Domingo, UNICEF/ONAPLAN.

TANNAHILL, R. (1980) *Sex in History*, New York, Stein & Day Publishers.

TRAVIN, S. and PROTTER, B. (1993) *Sexual Perversion*, New York, Plenum Press.

TRIMMER, R. (Ed.) (1978) *The Visual Dictionary of Sex*, New York, Pan Books.

WEINBERG, M. S. (Ed.) (1976) *Sex Research: Studies from the Kinsey Institute*, New York, Oxford University Press.

ZINICK, G. (1985) 'Identity Conflict or Adaptive Flexibility? Bisexuality Reconsidered', in KLEIN, F. and WOLF, T. (Eds) *Two Lives to Lead: Bisexuality in Men and Women*, New York, Harrington Park Press.

## Chapter 8

# Male Bisexuality in Peru and the Prevention of AIDS

*Carlos F. Cáceres*

Over the last decade, so-called Latin American bisexuality has become a focus of interest among epidemiologists and public health practitioners. Needless to say, this is connected to the growth of an AIDS epidemic initially affecting men who were reported as 'homosexuals' in most countries' surveillance reports in the region, an expansion that has paid attention neither to fixed borders of gender nor attributed sexual orientations, nor to the sexual identities that had somehow been assumed to govern the epidemic's growth. As World Health Organization (WHO) statistics show, the proportion of reported cases of AIDS among women in Latin America is steadily increasing, which tends to be explained by a growing transmission of HIV from bisexual men to their female partners. The male-to-female case ratio had fallen from 6.9 in 1987 to 4.8 in 1993 (PAHO, 1993).

A simple criticism of this account might stress the ethical problems posed by public health authorities' uncritical acceptance of the epidemic as essentially a homosexual plague, and their further construction of bisexuality as a bridge connecting an infected (and infectious) constituency to the 'general population', that is, as a population 'risk factor' for AIDS: an account in which bisexuals become intrinsically evil people. From a sexual health perspective, such reasoning encourages a reinforcement of traditional techniques of social control regarding sexuality. This is well illustrated in the energies physicians have devoted (and continue to devote) to the identification of the 'bisexual connection', assumed as an almost necessary explanation of female HIV infections (particularly in countries where injecting drug use is rare). In what some could call Foucauldian terms, the physician's role as instrumental to the gaze and the knowledge/power of traditional sexual ideology when interviewing someone with AIDS is not all that distant from the role that a priest or an attorney would adopt in analogous circumstances. From the standpoint of intervention development, this framing not only creates obstacles for solidarity and support, but has commonly led to programmatic inertia, as it has not *per se* led to any decrease in the number of risky, unprotected sexual acts between potentially infected partners.

Indeed, public health approaches to this characterization of bisexuality have not been useful. On the one hand, a simplistic biomedical model, which considers essentially two, or maybe three clusters of men (namely, homosexuals, heterosexuals and bisexuals) with clearly separated social referents and lifestyles, does not match a 'real world' in which most people are anything but unequivocally identified with a particular way of life or sexual self-image. Only men who self-identify as homosexual (or gay) – that is, a rather small proportion of homosexually active men in Latin America – have been targeted by AIDS prevention messages by local NGOs involved in AIDS prevention in the gay community. Most others, and the women who have sex with them, have usually been bombarded with a communicational fantasy of heterosexual love and fidelity as a solution to the risks of AIDS, while condom use has been offered as a second-class measure for those who are 'promiscuous'. Not specifically addressed by any of these approaches, behaviourally bisexual men who are not gay-identified tend to embrace by default the fantasy of heterosexuality, with allied implications for AIDS prevention.

On the other hand, naive culturalist critiques of such models tend to overstress cultural or subcultural differences, to assume foreign social structures to be the result of internal stabilization processes that should be accepted as such, and to suggest they correspond to cognitive processes that are totally incompatible to 'ours'. In this context, more attention is given to the representation of an essentially static social universe, and the rhetorical power of its internal logic, than to the search for avenues of change. In the same way as 'African promiscuity' (Watney, 1991), Latin American bisexuality may have been regarded as a rarity that determines the fortune of the region's population in relation to the AIDS epidemic.

Little has been written so far about the evolving, coexisting discourses about sexuality and gender that influence, rather than determine, interpersonal and micro-social interactions and, ultimately, behaviours. Simon and Gagnon's theory of sexual scripts (Simon and Gagnon, 1984), along with the more general constructionist and symbolic interactionist approaches, is useful in this respect. According to this theory, sexual reality is determined at three interrelated levels. The *cultural scenario* constitutes the level of unquestioned hegemonic discourses on sexuality, which experience varying degrees of contradiction from alternative counter-hegemonic projects. *Interpersonal scripts* may either reproduce the mandates of the cultural scenario or allow for re-elaborations in terms of each participant's specific interpretations and personal positions with regard to hegemonic discourses. Finally, *intra-psychic scripts* represent the final *loci* of resistance where individuals confront their interpretations of the cultural mandates with their desires and behaviours, thus negotiating sexual identities and reconstructing self-images. In a recent paper, Laumann, Gagnon and Michael (1994) elaborate on this earlier framework, introducing structural factors such as social class, geography, ethnicity and age as additional determinants of sexual scripts, framing them within the perspective of sexual networks.

A consideration of cultural scenarios in relation to bisexuality is useful. In many cases, homosexual sex may be referred to not as sex but as 'having fun', 'messing around' (Aggleton, 1993). In this respect, and in the case of Latin America, it helps to realize that 'bisexual' (or 'bisexuality') is not a meaningful category for most people. At least, it is not a category with normative meaning. A strong body of data supports the notion that, in most Latin cultures, the question 'What is the biological sex of the person with whom you have sex?' is far less important than 'Who is the *man* there?', meaning either *who looks more like the man* or *who does what men do*. That is, having sex with a biological man is right as long as you are the *man* involved (Carrier, 1985; Parker, 1987, 1991, 1994; Alonso and Koreck, 1989; Parker and Carballo, 1990; Tielman, Carballo and Hendriks, 1991; Guimaraes, 1994; Cáceres and Cortiñas, in press).

At the same time, both the interpersonal and the intra-psychic levels offer a space in which the erotic is elaborated as a set of discourses of resistance to hegemonic sexuality and gender structures (Parker, 1991). It is not necessary to use biological explanations of homoeroticism to account for it; the role of prohibition probably has as much influence in the construction of hetero-sexual desire as it does in the generation of homosexual desire.

In consequence, we need better views of the hierarchies in which people organize these discourses (cultural scenarios) and strategically negotiate the personal and social meanings of their desires and behaviours according to such hierarchies (interpersonal and intra-psychic scripts). Factors operating at each of these three levels are likely to be linked intimately to the personal and social meanings of sexual risk-taking as defined from an AIDS perspective. In order to improve efficency, prevention programmes must have their starting point in new understandings of sexual cultural universes, and utilize the *loci* of resistance and agency they allow for.

The role of homoeroticism in the cultural construction of masculinity in urban Latin America needs close scrutiny. Based on preliminary information from on-going research in Lima, Peru, this chapter will examine important scripts of unprotected male bisexual behaviour in an attempt to identify obstacles to safer practice, and to suggest revisions to the public health mes-sages directed to each of the actors involved, in a way that empowers both men and women to remove some of the barriers to HIV prevention and social change.

## A Taxonomy of Homosexually Active Characters in Lima

While a post-modern consciousness may find taxonomies less than useful in the assumed context of fluid identities and styles, of blurred delimitations and complex determinations, they have practical value in allowing the construc-tion of partial, conditioned, temporary representations of reality that allow and support directioned action (Haraway, 1991). This is the use to which they will be put here.

In a study of sexual behaviour among men who were having sex with men (MSM) carried out in Lima in 1992, we offered a list of labels from which respondents could choose one for self-description (Cáceres and Rosasco, 1992). Terms included were: homosexual, gay, bisexual, heterosexual, transsexual, *travesti*, woman, and other. Interestingly, choosing homosexual/gay versus bisexual or heterosexual did not depend on sexual behaviour (i.e. whether it had been exclusively homosexual versus bisexual) during the past year. Additionally, this proved one of the most difficult questions for subjects to answer, and people's doubts made us realize that difficulties arose from the obviously diverse meanings and stigmas they had learned to assign to the same words. While the term 'gay' might mean more feminine and/or vulgar for some, it might signify a more modern, proud and/or macho person for others. 'Homosexual' was a sober and technical term for some, while others felt it offensive. Our question failed to reveal the inner truth about frequencies of sexual identities in this population, but showed us how meaningless our system was for many people, to the extent that subgroups within our sample seemed to have learned different – sometimes contradictory – meanings for those terms. Moreover, the sets of possible identities each respondent had perceived as available were experientially diverse, as were the ways each resolved the dilemma of choosing a label depending on what they thought they did or were.

On the basis of these data, we began to construct a conceptual model that could explain better the diversity of experience among MSM in Lima, and a model that could be used in the design and sampling process for our current research. Within this model, the lifestyles of homosexually active men in metropolitan Lima seem to vary across at least the following axes:

- Social class, which is a strong determinant of social networks, thus influencing life chances. Middle-class experience in particular is linked to a whole array of specific bodily codes and conceptions of privacy, intimacy and propriety, and also regulates access to international travel and consequently to the influence of foreign sexual cultures (although increasingly less due to the mass-mediated globalization of Anglo/European culture).
- Degree and patterns of sexual involvement with women, which correspond to conventional biomedical categories describing the orientation of sexual behaviour.
- Activity/passivity (i.e. sexual compliance with dominant sexual/gender norms), related to whether or not a man, regardless of his partner's gender, acts sexually *as a man* (that is, whether he is *activo* or not). Being *activo* with another man does not harm his self-image or his public image as a man.
- Conventional virility/femininity (i.e. generic compliance with dominant sexual/gender norms), related to whether or not a man, regardless of his partner's sex, behaves socially as a man (in other words, whether or not he adopts conventional masculine behaviour in his diverse non-sexual interactions with others, including dress, ways of walking or speaking, intonation, vocabulary, etc.).

- Sexual self-image or identity, related to a particular person's self-reflection on whether or not her/his experience is compatible with a specific sexual identity among those s/he has identified as possible, on the basis of perceived social values.
- Participation in sex-for-profit exchanges, since more or less overt patterns of exchange determine variable patterns of sexual behaviour and identity. More formal exchanges are usually linked to specific identities, which are at least temporary and imply regular contact with particular sexual subcultures.
- Age, as related to historically evolving processes of construction of (homo)sexuality in people's experience (including people's desires, perceived norms regarding those desires, and possible adoption of a negotiated sexual identity among those populating the perceived sexual universe), as well as to concrete sexual networks.
- Degree of participation in homosexual subculture(s), as connected to variable degrees of acculturation into alternative worldviews that imply different ways of socializing, networking, self-identifying sexually, understanding and valuing diverse sexual practices and, possibly, reacting politically against hegemonic sexual norms (e.g. engaging in gay activism versus, say, adopting a closeted pattern of homosexual experience).

In an on-going study, we asked male adolescents and young adults to make free lists of terms related to men who had sex with other men. Later, we requested them to sort cards with thirty such terms. A similar exercise was undertaken with young men known to have sex with other men. A preliminary analysis suggests that the structure of the lists elicited through this procedure differed across groups, and that when the same terms were sorted by people of the two groups, important differences emerged, not only in relation to the meanings assigned to terms pertaining to specific gay subcultures or to the hegemonic macho cultural system, but also with regard to attitudes and value judgments subsumed in the use of identical terms across both groups.

For example, free lists provided by 'general group' adolescents included terms such as *maricon, cabro, resquete* and others which were not elicited from MSM becuase of their strongly pejorative meaning. Evidence of this emerged in sorting, where these terms were sorted together by MSM and labelled as *incorrect words referred to homosexuality*. Similarly, the word *moderno*, which within the gay subculture suggests role versatility (see below), did not have this second meaning for the general group, who understand the term in its overt meaning of *modern*. *Homosexual*, however, is an example of a term that for subgroups in both the general group and that of MSM may be assigned either the aseptic connotation of a scientific term or the pejorative strength of an insult, the differences being related probably to the uses of this word in particular social networks. In summary, subcultures of MSM seem to have (re)created semantic systems in which some words are invented, assigned second (cryptic) meanings, or transformed in their value connotations, a process which is far from uniform and shows differences from the parlance of the general group.

On the basis of informal interviews with key informants, a taxonomy was developed and discussed in focus group sessions of young men who had sex with other men, thus allowing for subsequent adjustment. A constellation of characters emerged, as described later. It must be noted that any such 'characters' should not be seen as neatly defined nor as static. Some of them may constitute social actors in the process of extinction, whereas others are only just emerging.

This constellation should therefore be seen as a snapshot of events within an on-going struggle for meaning, as an on-going negotiation of the peculiarities of a cultural system that governs the heterogeneity of homoerotic desire/ practice and its interpretations among a fraction of men in urban Lima, including issues such as the emergence of new possibilities of linkage between desires and lifestyles. Again, this taxonomy is contingent to an historical context, as is the case everywhere, particularly in countries outside the developed West (see Altman, 1994; Tan, 1994), and bears a strong relationship to a process of cultural globalization through the expansion of communication and travel. It is also permeated by numerous social phenomena such as those related to class and ethnic prejudice.[1] Our working sexual constellation involves the characters described below.

### Men from Working-Class Backgrounds

The *activo, mostacero* or *cacanero* (equivalent to the *Mayate* in Mexico) is a macho character who does not consider his heterosexuality to be questioned by occasional sexual involvement with *cabros* or *travestis*. Some sort of benefit (usually money, beer or a gift) is assumed by his peers to have been obtained from his homosexual transactions. He is not supposed to experience desire for male sexual partners, as he is assumed to be attracted only (and always) to women. However, as *mostaceros* function as a sort of reservoir of manhood, their sexual responsiveness, when appropriately stimulated, is supposed to be natural and inevitable. Their sexual exchanges are supposed to rigidly replicate the mandates of sexual/gender norms. They will be insertive in both oral and anal sex, without ever thinking of even touching their partners' genitals. Should they do this to a *cabro*, the latter would consider them to be *estafadores* (cheaters) who are not 'real men', and their peers would think they were becoming *cabros* as well. In spite of the fact that they are aware of AIDS, *machos latinos* use condoms inconsistently. As they consider AIDS a gay disease, they do not feel themselves at risk. The female partners of *mostaceros*, both of a 'permanent' (i.e. girlfriends, spouses) or occasional sort, usually accept their male partners' involvement with other people, and do not question the normality of their own unprotected sexual encounters with them. This character may be said to be in a process of dilution and expansion in the common-sense sexual knowledge and practical possibilities of most working-class adolescents and young adults.

The *cabro* or *marica* (equivalent to the traditional faggot in Anglo popular culture), is a character who is effeminate and usually does not call himself a man, and whose sexual desire is oriented towards *mostaceros*. He will usually engage only in receptive oral and/or anal sex, and may not like a macho sexual partner to touch his genitals. He usually participates in the ghettoized gay subculture of working-class neighbourhoods, and tends to dismiss the need for protection with *mostaceros*, as he considers them to be at much lower risk of HIV. This character is probably in the process of extinction, giving rise to a working-class version of a gay man.

The *travesti* is a man who cross-dresses, usually permanently, and performs what has been called a mock femininity (i.e. manners that largely exaggerate the feminine norm, and sexual aggressiveness). He will usually engage only in receptive oral and/or anal sex, though, particularly in the context of prostitution, he may be sought as a versatile or an only-insertive partner. He also participates in a sexual subculture that tends to be violent and marginal, yet in many cases *travestis* are integrated into working-class neighbourhood communities as hairdressers and cooks, and develop friendships with local women. It is as hairdressers that many of them have sex with young men adopting a *mostacero* role, including many 'first-timers'. However, the easiest and best paid economic activity for a *travesti* is street prostitution. In spite of being 'fake women', *travestis* become objects of desire for working-class men. As an example of what Parker (1991) calls the structure of the erotic (in opposition to gender and sexuality norms), the public discourse of disapproval coexists with some relatively acceptable statements regarding their irresistible femininity, which suggest that it is only natural for a 'real man' to like them. In fact, *travesti* prostitutes usually constitute an exotic speciality that many working-class men actively look for. They embody a key transgressive erotic object of the local culture of desire. Protected sex is neither extensive nor consistent among *travestis*, which may be linked to their concern to hide their male genitals in sex work, as clients may expect them to pretend they are 'real women'.

## Among Men from Upper-Class and Middle-Class Backgrounds

The *entendido* (translated literally as *connoisseur*) is a man in his twenties or thirties who knows the middle-class gay scene to some extent. He likes women and tends to be socially and sexually involved with them. He does not see himself as a different sort of man. However, he acknowledges to diverse degrees his attraction to other men, and will frequently engage in same-gender sex with either friends or occasional partners, often after consuming alcohol. When he is comfortable enough, he will talk about his encounters as *vacilones* (having fun) to a few selected friends. His sexual practices and the roles he adopts cover a wide variety of possibilities across the activity/passivity axis. His awareness of STD risks with men is variable, and is usually impaired by alcohol. Protection during homosexual sex is, consequently, variable, yet more infrequent than in the case of working-class men who are *mostaceros*. Protection with regular female partners is infrequent. Current (as compared to former) *entendidos* tend to be more versatile sexually and more open about their 'having fun'.

The *married bisexual* is, in our taxonomy, a man who marries a woman principally for social desirability reasons, as essentially he is attracted to other men. Sex with their wives remains unprotected as mutual fidelity is assumed. The prevalence of this character is probably in decline.

The *gay-identified bisexual* is, conversely, a man who is attracted to women and gets sexually involved with them, but who is also attracted to and sexually active with other men. He should be differentiated from *façade bisexuals*, men attracted to and active with men only or mostly, who choose to self-present themselves as bisexuals as a strategy of partial transaction with the norm. The gay-identified bisexual participates in the gay scene to diverse degrees and self-identifies as gay or bisexual. His sexual repertoire tends to be broad and safe with both men and women. This species is new in the local sexuality/gender panorama, and results from the influence of first-world metropolis' gay culture in the media and in travellers.

Among men who usually do not have sex with women, the *gay man* is the typical man who assumes a gay lifestyle and participates in the local gay scene. The traditional closet of the past is becoming less frequent. Of varied sexual practices, he is increasingly *moderno*, that is, both receptive and insertive. He is very knowledgeable about AIDS and regularly safe in occasional sex, though not uncommonly unsafe in steady relationships. Rather than macho types as it was in the past, his sexual ideal is turning out to be somebody like him, and he is increasingly more masculine and concerned with his own masculine looks (i.e. he adopts a model of gayness that stresses the assertion of masculinity, as described by Tan (1994) and Altman (1994).

### Commercial Homosexual Activity

Players of all characters from the working-class sectors (and some of those from the middle-class sectors) engage in sex-for-profit exchanges. The common name given to a wide range of such characters when they function as providers of commercial sex is *flete*. Male prostitution is generally called *fleteo*. *Travestis* are an exception, and they are referred to through mention of the streets where they work (e.g. Arequipa Avenue *travestis*).

The fantasy of material interest is usually played with by all working-class *mostaceros* in their homosexual encounters with feminized characters (*cabros* and *travestis*), as they usually see themselves as doing a favour to them. However, more organized prostitution systems imply their physical displacement to red light spots of the city where direct contacts are made and an economic deal is usually reached before any sexual service is provided (in a way similar to that described for Mexico, the Philippines or Morocco by Izazola (1993), Tan (1994) and Boushaba *et al.* (1994), respectively). In such cases, a new identity (i.e. a *flete* identity) may emerge, which involves a relative tolerance of sexual practices regarded as unmanly, and is associated with an anxiety to meet new clients that at times looks like a strong interest in being picked up, and a taste for types and looks of clients as well as cars' brand names. It is possible that, for some *fletes*, the fascination of interactions otherwise unthinkable across barriers of age and social class represents the major motive to experiment with *fleteo* or continue such practice. At the same time, most new *fletes* try to maintain a reputation of being *activos* among their peers in red light spots, although many become versatile in the intimacy of interaction with clients.

Some working-class *cabros* and, increasingly, middle-class *entendidos* and gay men, participate in *fleteo*, though the latter may be inclined to choose bars or telephonic services for their contacts, rather than the streets. The higher their socio-economic background, the more likely it is that their motives for getting involved in *fleteo* will include a search of personal fun, emotion and curiosity about marginal forms of sexual expression. Most *fletes* say they practise safer sex and consider their clients to be equally interested in safety.

The situation is different with *travestis*. Transvestite prostitution takes place in a context of constant violence and marginality, and safe sex concerns are, understandably, far less salient. Additionally, many clients tend to pay more if condoms are not used, which constitutes an offer difficult to decline.

### Possibilities for Action

As described, bisexual involvements take place in quite diverse contexts in Lima, and are structured by social class, self-image, sexual and generic subjection to dominant sexual/gender norms, age, participation in homosexual subcultures, and involvement in commercial sex. From the perspective of HIV prevention, each context offers a particular configuration of HIV-related risk for the actors involved. This is determined by HIV prevalence in their social/sexual networks, their sexual practices and roles, and the prevalence of a consistently safe sexual praxis in both homosexual and heterosexual encounters.

Those at highest risk continue to be men holding the most traditional roles in the working classes, namely *mostaceros*, *travestis* and *cabros*, and the female partners of the former. *Mostaceros* need prevention programmes in which the myth of AIDS as a disease of others is finally destroyed, and in which safe sex is presented as a protection for their partners, be they women or men.

Their female partners need to develop skills to evaluate their spouses' sexual activity outside their relationship, and to negotiate the possibility of barrier protection, which is indeed a difficult task. This should be achieved in the context of broader women's health programmes, focusing, for example, on STDs more generally.

Regarding *travestis*, the extreme conditions of marginality which surround transvestite prostitution and reduce possibilities of prevention should be faced and modified. To a lesser extent, *married bisexuals* and some *entendidos* from the middle classes who engage in unsafe sex, as a result, perhaps, of low self-esteem or alcohol use, need to be reached by communication strategies that offer them basic support and opportunities for change in the confidential context they will require. As they cannot be reached in a ghetto setting, mass media channels or outreach programmes in cruising areas may perhaps be successful. Assertiveness and open communication regarding the possibilities of sex outside the relationship should be promoted among the women who may be female partners of such men.

Finally, the condom (and, eventually, the Femidom, or female condom) needs to be eroticized. To the extent that both men and women begin to associate good sex with condoms and these are naturalized as something intrinsically erotic, barrier protection will become more prevalent in both homo and heterosexual encounters.

### Conclusions

The depictions of bisexuality described here correspond to a partial vision of male bisexuality in Lima in the late 1980s and early 1990s. As mentioned before, they reflect the inconsistencies of research in progress and the contradictions inherent in what we call reality. They provide, however, an illustration of what can be achieved by the kind of research into representations of sexuality that is becoming popular among many AIDS prevention researchers.

They probably resemble what could be found in urban areas of many other countries in Latin America, with only some changes in terms, as Parker (1991) in Brazil and Izazola (1993) in Mexico, among others, have shown. We are sure that knowledge of these representations is important for the design and implementation of programmes that take into account the heterogeneity of sexual meanings and the pre-eminence of cultural diversity (Parker, 1994). This kind of research has the potential to identify avenues of resistance to traditional ideologies and practices connected to current sexual risks, and may point the way towards more sexually democratic AIDS prevention (and sexual health promotion) programmes in the 1990s.

**Note**

This chapter describes research conducted with the support of research/ training grants from AIDSTECH/FHI, the Fogarty International Center, and the Ford Foundation.

1 An example of this can be seen in the contested meanings of 'gay'. The hegemonic working-class meaning of 'gay' offers a perhaps more tolerant way of describing both *cabros* and *travestis*. Among members of the middle class, the term has both this working-class sense and that of a more modern gayness. Similarly, whereas for *cabros* and *travestis*, gay might refer to closeted middle-class homosexuals, middle-class gay men adopt the term with no regrets. Finally, gay activists tend to perceive a traditional activist content in the term, in relation to a proud self-consciousness of constituency and lifestyle.

**References**

AGGLETON, P. (1993) 'Sexual Behaviour Research and HIV/AIDS', paper given at the VIIIth International Conference on AIDS in Africa, Marrakech.

ALONSO, A. and KORECK, M. (1989) 'Silences: "Hispanics", AIDS and Sexual Practices', *Differences*, 1, pp. 101–24.

ALTMAN, D. (1994) 'The Invention of Gay as a Global Category', unpublished manuscript, Melbourne, Australia.

BOUSHABA, A., ALI, H. and IMANE, L. (1994) 'Prevention Proximity among Male Sex Workers in Casablanca and Marrakesh', *Abstracts Book, Xth International Conference on AIDS*, Yokohama, Japan.

CÁCERES, C. and CORTIÑAS, J. (in press) 'Fantasy Island: Alcohol and Gender Roles in a Latino Gay Bar', *Journal of Alcohol and Drug Issues*.

CÁCERES, C. and ROSASCO, A. (1992) 'Determinants of Risk Behaviour among Men Who Have Sex with Men in Lima', *Abstracts Book, VIIIth International Conference on AIDS*, Amsterdam, The Netherlands.

CARRIER, J. (1985) 'Mexican Male Bisexuality', *Journal of Homosexuality*, 11, pp. 75–85.

GUIMARAES, C. (1994) 'A bissexualidade masculina e os riscos da transmissao do HIV', oral presentation at the seminar AIDS, Saúde Reprodutiva e Políticas Públicas, Rio de Janeiro.

HARAWAY, D. (1991) *Simians, Cyborgs and Women: The Reinvention of Nature*, London and New York, Routledge.

LAUMANN, E., GAGNON, J. and MICHAEL, R. (1994) 'A Sociological Perspective on Sexual Action', in PARKER, R. and GAGNON, J. (Eds) *Conceiving Sexuality: Approaches to Sex Research in a Postmodern World*, London and New York, Routledge.

PAN AMERICAN HEALTH ORGANIZATION (1993) *AIDS Epidemiological Surveillance in the Americas*, Quarterly Report, June.

PARKER, R. (1987) 'Acquired Immunodeficiency Syndrome in Urban Brazil', *Medical Anthropology Quarterly*, 1, pp. 155–75.

PARKER, R. (1991) *Bodies, Pleasures and Passions: Sexual Culture in Contemporary Brazil*, Boston, Beacon Press.

PARKER, R. (1994) 'Sexual Cultures, HIV Transmission and AIDS Prevention', *AIDS*, 8 (suppl. 1), pp. S309–S314.

PARKER, R. and CARBALLO, M. (1990) 'Qualitative Research on Homosexual and Bisexual Behaviour Relevant to HIV/AIDS', *Journal of Sex Research*, 27, pp. 497–525.

SIMON, M. and GAGNON, J. (1984) 'Sexual Scripts', *Society*, 22, pp. 53–60.

TAN, M. (1994) 'From Bakla to Gay: Shifting Gender Identities and Sexual Behaviours among Filipino Men Who Have Sex with Men', in PARKER, R. and GAGNON, J. (Eds) *Conceiving Sexuality: Approaches to Sex Research in a Postmodern World*, London and New York, Routledge.

TIELMAN, R., CARBALLO, M. and HENDRIKS, A. (Eds) (1991) *Bisexuality and HIV/AIDS*, Buffalo, Promethius Press.

WATNEY, S. (1991) 'Missionary Positions, AIDS and Africa', *Critical Quarterly*, 31, 3, pp. 45–62.

WORLD HEALTH ORGANIZATION (1994) *The HIV/AIDS Pandemic: 1994 Overview*, Geneva, WHO.

## Chapter 9

# Bisexuality and HIV/AIDS in Brazil

*Richard G. Parker*

Although bisexual behaviour appears to have played a role in HIV transmission in a number of different countries, it has been described as especially important in shaping the HIV/AIDS epidemic in Brazil, the country with the highest number of reported cases of AIDS in the Latin American region, and one of the most potentially explosive HIV/AIDS epidemics anywhere in the world (see Daniel and Parker, 1991, 1993; Parker and Tawil, 1991; Parker *et al.*, 1994). While early epidemiological reports from throughout the country focused on HIV transmission principally in relation to men with exclusively homosexual behaviour, high numbers of AIDS cases were recorded as well among men reporting sexual relations not only with other men, but also with women. During the first decade of the AIDS epidemic in Brazil, for example, roughly 20 per cent of the reported cases of AIDS in Brazil were classified as bisexual males (Rodrigues and Chequer, 1989), and it has been suggested that at least some cases of AIDS classified as the result of heterosexual transmission might in fact be behaviourally bisexual men who, due to social stigma and discrimination associated with homosexual practices, might have failed to report their same-sex sexual contacts (Castilho *et al.*, 1989).

While data on HIV seroprevalence, as opposed to reported cases of AIDS, have been limited in Brazil, they have tended to confirm the general picture presented in analyses based on AIDS case reporting. One early study of fifty-eight behaviourally bisexual men in Rio de Janeiro, for example, found a seroprevalence rate of 28 per cent for HIV-1 and 7 per cent for HTLV-I (Côrtes *et al.*, 1989). A contemporary study of 131 female sexual partners of bisexual men, also conducted in Rio de Janeiro, reported a seropositive rate of 25 per cent among those women who reported engaging in vaginal intercourse and 62 per cent among those who reported anal as well as vaginal sex (Sion *et al.*, 1989).

On the basis of such limited data, it has been frequently suggested in both the popular media and the scientific literature that bisexual behaviour may serve as a kind of epidemiological 'bridge' between supposedly high prevalence populations (such as exclusively homosexual males) and low prevalence groups (such as heterosexual females and males). Indeed, on a number of occasions, leading clinicians and AIDS researchers have characterized a kind of stereotypic 'bisexual male' as one of the principal villains of the epidemic

– almost wilfully responsible, through his largely clandestine sexual behaviour, for the infection of his innocent female partners and, by extension, their children.

The social and economic factors influencing changes in relative rates of HIV transmission, and the rapid increase in heterosexual transmission that has undeniably taken place in Brazil in recent years, are clearly more complex and varied than this characterization would suggest. While bisexual behaviour may be one factor influencing rates of heterosexual transmission, the fact of the matter is that such behaviour has actually been far more frequently commented or speculated upon than investigated or understood. This general lack of understanding, together with frequent prejudice and discrimination, has in turn raised a number of difficult dilemmas for AIDS prevention activities, and has made it exceptionally difficult to respond to the spread of HIV infection through AIDS education programmes and interventions designed to serve the needs of behaviourally bisexual men and their sexual partners, whether male or female (Parker, 1988, 1990, 1994; Daniel and Parker, 1991, 1993; Parker *et al.*, 1994).

This chapter seeks to provide an overview of the social organization of male bisexual behaviour in Brazil, and of its relation to the HIV/AIDS epidemic. It will review existing knowledge, drawn, in particular, from anthropological and sociological research on homosexuality and bisexuality in the social and cultural context of contemporary Brazilian life. In addition, it will briefly discuss empirical data collected in Rio de Janeiro on bisexual behaviour and the risk of HIV transmission. Finally, it will seek to explore the implications of existing data for the development of further research and the elaboration of more effective intervention and education strategies aimed at reducing the spread of HIV/AIDS.

### The Social Construction of Bisexual Behaviour

The role of bisexual behaviour in the dynamics of HIV transmission in Brazil has posed a number of problems for existing epidemiological models or paradigms. In light of social and behavioural research carried out over an extended period on patterns of sexual behaviour in Brazil, however, the importance of bisexuality comes as little surprise. Indeed, long before the emergence of the AIDS epidemic, anthropologists and sociologists working in both rural and urban Brazil had pointed to an important pattern of sexual interaction in which occasional, or even frequent, same-sex sexual interactions between men need not necessarily call into question male gender identity (see Fry, 1982, 1985; Parker, 1985). The implications of this pattern for the social organization of homosexual and bisexual behaviour, and the relations between such behaviour, HIV transmission and AIDS prevention, have recently been explored in some detail (see, in particular, Daniel and Parker, 1993).

A fuller understanding of many of these issues depends upon a sense of how relatively recent, and, at some level, how superficial, notions such as 'homosexuality' and 'heterosexuality' are in Brazilian culture. While cultural categories such as *'homossexualidade'* and *'heterossexualidade'* are certainly present in Brazil, and have in fact become increasingly common terms in the language of everyday life, particularly with the emergence of HIV and AIDS, they are nonetheless not necessarily the most important or salient classifications used to structure the sexual universe in daily life. On the contrary, categories such as *homossexualidade* and *heterossexualidade* have traditionally been less significant than notions such as *'atividade'* ('activity') and *'passividade'* ('passivity'), which are understood both as distinct roles within the sexual act and as profoundly different manifestations of masculinity and femininity (see Fry, 1982, 1985; Parker, 1989, 1991, 1994; Daniel and Parker, 1993).

Given this focus on activity and passivity as key coordinates of the sexual universe, the object (whether female or male) of one's sexual desire may well be less significant in the subjective construction of one's sexual identity than is the role performed in one's sexual interactions. Particularly among members of lower classes, for whom more elite medical and scientific categories such as homosexuality or bisexuality are perhaps particularly distant, the so-called active (insertive) partners in same-sex interactions do not necessarily consider themselves to be either *'homossexual'* ('homosexual') or *'bissexual'* ('bisexual'), and their equally 'active' interactions with members of the opposite sex, or their social roles as husbands or fathers, may be more significant in the constitution of their own sense of self than are the occasional sexual relations they may have with other males (see Fry, 1982, 1985; Parker, 1989, 1991, 1994; Daniel and Parker, 1993).

This is not to say that active/passive role separation among men who have sex with men in Brazil is necessarily absolute or exclusive. On the contrary, relatively high erotic value is placed upon a certain flexibility in sexual encounters, a willingness to transgress rules and prohibitions (see Parker, 1989, 1991, 1994; Daniel and Parker, 1993), and this is no less true in the dynamics of sexual activity and passivity than in any other area. Indeed, research findings on homosexual and bisexual behaviour among men in Rio de Janeiro, for example, suggest that active/passive role exchange may occur rather frequently – particularly when compared with other Latin societies (Parker *et al.*, 1991b; Parker, 1994). The ideological structures that distinguish between activity and passivity, while simultaneously opening up possibilities for the transgression of this distinction, however, thus create a social and cultural context in which the constitution of sexual and gender identities can easily find what might be described as points of escape within the system itself – contradictory or parallel meanings which make it possible for the assumption of unwanted or socially undesirable characteristics (such as male 'passivity' or, more recently, 'homosexuality') to be avoided or ignored. An active partner in same-sex as well as opposite-sex interactions can thus relatively easily ignore his homosexual behaviours, while the active partner who is also occasionally passive can choose to disregard his passivity, and so on. Sexual identities may thus be situationally contingent – depending upon the specific circumstances, one sexual identity may be chosen over others. In a different situation, the choice may also be different. The constitution of one's sexual identity (or identities) must necessarily be negotiated in the flow of social interaction, and interaction, in turn, is necessarily shaped by the specific contexts or situations in which it takes place (see Parker, 1991, 1994; Daniel and Parker, 1993).

As might be expected given this emphasis on changing situations and negotiation, a number of distinct sexual subcultures (interacting networks of individuals sharing a similar set of cultural meanings and assumptions – a similar cultural grammar) developed around same-sex interactions have become increasingly evident in urban Brazilian life, particularly in recent decades. Yet the boundaries of these subcultures have been considerably more flexible than seems to be the case in the gay communities of the United States or many parts of Western Europe, where a more clearly defined gay community has emerged. The majority of these same-sex subcultures in most major Brazilian cities have been focused less on a shared sense of sexual identity than on the search for sexual partners and the diverse play of sexual desires, and a wide range of sexual 'types' have tended to intermingle within the space of these subcultures: effeminate '*bichas*' (which might be translated into English more or less as 'queens'), highly masculine '*bofes*' (which might be translated as 'studs' or 'trade'), '*michês*' ('hustlers'), '*travestis*' ('transvestites'), and '*entendidos*' (perhaps the most general and all-encompassing category, which literally refers to 'those who know' the rules of this social universe, and functions more or less like the notion of 'gay' in English, though perhaps without the same political connotations of the English-language term), to name just a few of the most common sexual categories.

Over time, the shape of these different subcultures has clearly changed, at least in part as a response to the evolving HIV/AIDS epidemic itself. Particularly among the middle class, though also increasingly among the lower classes, a notion of gay identity and a sense of community similar to that found in the gay communities of many developed countries has increasingly begun to emerge, with its own institutions (bars, discos, theatres, gay organizations, and so on) and its own social events (especially organized parties either at private homes or, more recently, at gay clubs or music halls). Entrance into and exit from this emerging community, however, continues to be relatively fluid, and the sexual classifications that take shape within it may well be transformed, or even cease to function, outside its particular boundaries (see Parker, 1989, 1994; Daniel and Parker, 1991, 1993).

This emphasis on changing situations and the negotiation of sexual meanings, on diverse sexual types or classifications and open-ended sexual subcultures, and on a rapidly changing system for the social organization of sexual communities, offers a relatively high degree of fluidity and flexibility in the constitution of sexual interactions. It has been especially important in shaping the spread of the AIDS epidemic in Brazil, with its high incidence of cases among behaviourally bisexual men and, more recently, its rapid increase of HIV infection among women (Daniel and Parker, 1993; Guimarães, 1994; Parker, 1994). At the same time, it has perhaps limited many of the most effective channels for the development of AIDS prevention activities, as it has offered little opportunity for the most common health promotion strategies aimed at targeting AIDS prevention messages to clearly defined and self-identified 'risk groups'. Precisely because many men who have sex with other men, as well as with women, fail to identify themselves as either *homossexual* or *bissexual*, AIDS education messages directed to these audiences have proved to be relatively limited in their potential impact (Daniel and Parker, 1993; Parker, 1994; Parker *et al.*, 1994).

### Bisexual Behaviour and the Risk of HIV Transmission

The problems posed for HIV/AIDS prevention by the social and cultural construction of same-sex practices in Brazil are accentuated, as well, by a lack of reliable data on the actual risk behaviours and AIDS-related knowledge, attitudes, and beliefs of behaviourally bisexual men. While anthropological and sociological research on sexual culture and sexual ideology has offered important insights into the structure of many same-sex interactions, and into the ways in which lived sexual experience often escapes the categories and classifications of much epidemiological thinking, it has generally provided a good deal less information on the actual incidence of sexual risk behaviours – or on the ways in which risk behaviour may be changing as a response to HIV/AIDS. Empirical studies of sexual behaviour in Brazil have been almost non-existent, and it is only very recently that social and behavioural research focusing on sexual behaviour in relation to HIV transmission and AIDS has been initiated in order to address such questions in Brazil (see Daniel and Parker, 1991, 1993; Parker, 1994; Parker *et al.*, 1991b, 1994).

This lack of data on sexual behaviour has been magnified, as well, by the difficulties that are inherent in sampling behavioural patterns such as bisexuality. As in much HIV/AIDS behavioural research, the construction of representative, random probability samples of gay or bisexual men, or, for that matter, injecting drug users, in Brazil as elsewhere, is essentially an impossible task. Whenever social stigma exists in relation to a given behavioural pattern, not only is there a chance that at least some (if not most) individuals sampled through statistically generalizable methods will hold back information concerning socially disapproved behaviours, but this is in fact very likely. Attempts to gather representative, population-based, data on questions such as the incidence of bisexual behaviour are thus fundamentally problematic, and much of what can be known about sexual risk behaviour among such populations must necessarily rely upon targeted sampling strategies that are inevitably limited by the options open for recruiting participants (see Turner *et al.*, 1989; Parker and Carballo, 1990, 1991; Parker *et al.*, 1991a).

Acknowledging such limitations, research carried out since 1989 in Rio de Janeiro nonetheless suggests that the incidence of high-risk sexual behaviours continues to be significant among homosexual and bisexual men in Brazil. Based on a convenience sample constructed through snowball or network sampling and targeted recruiting, a study of 503 homosexual and bisexual men carried out between October of 1989 and November of 1990, for example, suggests that high-risk behaviours continue to be practised by more than half the individuals interviewed – and that the incidence of risk behaviours is particularly high among those men who report sexual contact with both male and female partners (Parker, 1994; Parker *et al.*, 1991b, 1994).

While the focus of this study was to gather information on homosexual behaviour and behaviour change, and no special attempt was made to target behaviourally bisexual men, eighty-eight of the 503 men interviewed reported having engaged in sexual intercourse with female partners during a six-month period prior to being interviewed. Perhaps not surprisingly, given the social and cultural patterns described above, only 27 per cent of these men described themselves as 'bisexuals'. While nearly 14 per cent of these behaviourally bisexual men described themselves as 'homosexual' and another 2 per cent as 'gay,' 12 per cent described themselves employing some other classificatory category, and fully 44 per cent failed to respond at all (Parker, 1994; Parker *et al.*, 1991b).

Independent of the ways in which they classify their sexual identity or orientation, when asked about their knowledge of HIV/AIDS, the majority of the behaviourally bisexual sample showed a relatively high level of AIDS awareness (though less than was reported by the exclusively homosexual respondents). All eighty-eight had heard of AIDS, and 91 per cent reported that HIV is either definitely (75 per cent) or probably (16 per cent) transmitted through semen. Though with somewhat less certainty, nearly as many (89 per cent) reported that the use of condoms could definitely (50 per cent) or probably (39 per cent) reduce the sexual transmission of HIV. And although 23 per cent reported having made no changes in their sexual behaviour after having learned of AIDS, another 25 per cent reported having made some changes and 35 per cent reported having made major changes (Parker, 1994; Parker *et al.*, 1991b, 1994).

As important as these indications of AIDS awareness and self-reported behaviour change might potentially be, however, in turning to an examination of sexual practices it is apparent that high levels of risk behaviour continue to characterize a significant part of the sample. Relatively high incidence of insertive and, to a lesser extent, receptive anal intercourse were reported with male partners, for example, while condom use was reported to be relatively limited. While 75 per cent reported having anally penetrated another male in the previous six months, 57 per cent reported having done so without a condom, and while 41 per cent reported having been anally penetrated, 19 per cent reported having been penetrated without the use of a condom (Parker, 1994; Parker *et al.*, 1991b, 1994).

Perhaps not surprisingly, but certainly no less worrisome, the incidence of risk behaviours with female partners seems to be even more significant. Fully 56 per cent reported having engaged in anal intercourse with a female partner during the past six months, and 43 per cent reported having done so without the use of a condom. Of the 100 per cent of the sample reporting having engaged in vaginal intercourse during the six months prior to being interviewed, 89 per cent reported having done so without the use of a condom (Parker, 1994; Parker *et al.*, 1991b, 1994).

In short, then, within this limited sample of behaviourally bisexual men, risk behaviours continue to be practised with relative frequency, and condom use continues to be relatively limited. Patterns of risk behaviour can be found in relation to both male and female sexual partners, with even more signifi-cant levels of risk apparently characterizing heterosexual interactions, particu-larly due to the lower level of condom use in both anal and vaginal intercourse with women. The reasons for this continued practice of high-risk behaviours are of course multiple, and most probably vary depending on the specific situation in question. Among this particular sample, however, data suggest that complicated, and sometimes contradictory attitudes related to risk, sexual excitement, and condom use are clearly crucial. Of the men sampled, for example, 75 per cent classified anal penetration of another male without a condom as high-risk behaviour, while only 7 per cent considered it risky when using a condom. While 73 per cent classified anal penetration as highly exciting without a condom, however, only 23 per cent still considered it to be exciting when using a condom. Much the same association seems to hold true in relation to sex with women. Fifty-one per cent of the sample considered vaginal intercourse to be a high-risk activity without a condom, while only 6 per cent considered it risky with the use of a condom. While 76 per cent found vaginal intercourse highly exciting without a condom, however, only 35 per cent found it highly exciting when practised with the use of condoms (Parker, 1994; Parker *et al.*, 1991b, 1994).

These statistics suggest that the perception of risk may not always be enough to overcome a negative image of condom use as erotically unsatisfy-ing, regardless of the sexual practices or partners involved. Beyond this, however, they also suggest that even lower empirical rates of condom use with female partners than with male partners may be linked to a greater perception of risk in homosexual as opposed to heterosexual relations – a possibility that may well be accentuated, in turn, by the fear that condom use (associated in popular thought with AIDS, and hence with homosexuality) may also open up suspicions concerning the possibility of involvement in non-heterosexual be-haviour (Parker, 1994; Parker *et al.*, 1991b, 1994).

It is important to remember, of course, the limitations of these findings. While confirming many of the potential problems that may be posed by bisexual behaviour in relation to HIV/AIDS, and offering some insight into

possible questions that should be examined in greater depth, the only behavioural data thus far available concerning bisexuality in Brazil stem from a
limited, non-representative sample constructed in order to examine homosexual behaviour and behaviour change rather than bisexual behaviour. Precisely because much of the recruiting took place through homosexual
friendship networks, with no special effort to target bisexual men who may not
participate in such networks, the subsample of bisexual men within this population should not necessarily be considered typical. On the contrary, it is in all
likelihood characterized by higher levels of AIDS awareness and behavioural
risk reduction than would be the case with more socially isolated individuals
whose bisexual behaviours are more hidden or disconnected from the diverse
homosexual or gay subcultures that can be found in Rio de Janeiro. This, in
turn, should underline the urgent need for more extensive research focusing
on bisexual men and, whenever possible, on their female as well as male
sexual partners (Parker, 1994; Parker *et al.*, 1991b, 1994).

### AIDS Prevention for Behaviourally Bisexual Men

Taken together, the more qualitative research on the social and cultural
constitution of same-sex interactions that has been carried out over a number
of decades, along with the more quantitative investigation of homosexual and
bisexual behaviour initiated shortly after the emergence of AIDS, offer important background for assessing bisexual behaviour in relation to the risk of HIV
transmission in Brazil. In particular, these studies offer a number of insights
that might be useful in the design and implementation of AIDS prevention
programmes. At the same time, however, they also point to a number of
important issues that clearly must be examined in greater detail and among
a broader sample population in order to more effectively ground and, ultimately, evaluate information, education and prevention activities.

The ethnographic mapping of same-sex sexual subcultures in urban
centres such as Rio de Janeiro can clearly offer a point of departure for
segmenting and identifying points of access to the population of men who
have sex with men as well as with women. Sensitivity to the complexities
apparent in the categories and classifications used locally to distinguish different sexual types would suggest that somewhat distinct populations or subgroups should be approached in somewhat different ways. While *michês*,
*travestis, entendidos, bofes*, and the like may all exhibit bisexual behaviour at least
occasionally, the particularities of their different situations, and their identifiable association with different spaces within the sexual geography of the city,
suggest different intervention strategies. Programmes developed for male
prostitutes, for example, must clearly address the issue of bisexuality, but
within a framework in which a whole range of other issues (injecting drug use,
the power dynamics that may be involved in negotiating sexual practices
between members of different class or ethnic groups, and so on) may be

equally important. The same is of course true of programmes designed for men in institutional settings (such as prisons or the military), or for adolescent men involved in the process of exploring or acquiring their sexual identities. Precisely because multiple patterns of bisexual behaviour in fact exist, the specific AIDS prevention activities designed in response to these patterns must vary according to the needs of the populations involved (Parker and Carballo, 1991; Parker and Tawil, 1991).

On the basis of this kind of ethnographic understanding of sexual diversity in Brazil, however, it is also apparent that there exists a sizeable population of men who are uninvolved in any specific activities or situations (such as prostitution or institutional settings) that may result in bisexual behaviour, but who nonetheless actively seek out sexual interactions with other men as well as with women, often without the development of a distinct sexual identity or sense of sexual self as a result of these interactions. Precisely because of their relative lack of a distinct sexual identity, many of the important AIDS prevention activities developed for and by homosexual men and gay organizations, in Brazil as in many other societies, may largely fail to reach the population of behaviourally bisexual men, who clearly do not see themselves as the members of a distinct risk group, and who may or may not perceive the risks involved in their own sexual interactions, whether with other men or with women.

While these men are often extremely difficult to identify, and may indeed be likely to hide or even deny their same-sex interactions, access to them can nonetheless be achieved not only by targeting the undifferentiated mass of Brazilian males, but by focusing on a relatively limited number of relatively well-known geographic locations where same-sex interactions are sought out: specific parks, streets or plazas, certain cinemas, saunas, public toilets, and so on. Such locations are obviously sites in which a number of behaviourally distinct sub-populations intermingle – exclusively (and perhaps self-identified) homosexual males and behaviourally bisexual men mix together and interact in such settings in proportions and ways that are not yet fully understood.

Over the course of recent years, a range of different projects developed largely by community-based AIDS service organizations have sought to build upon such insights in developing interventions for specific groups of men who have sex with men in cities such as Rio de Janeiro and São Paulo. In Rio, for example, the Pegação Programme of outreach work targeting male prostitutes has been carried out in a number of sites since the early 1990s, and has been supported in part by the World Health Organization's Global Programme on AIDS, as well as by the Brazilian Ministry of Health's National AIDS Programme. In 1991 and 1992, with support from the USAID/Academy for Educational Development AIDSCOM Project, a local family-planning organization known as BEMFAM developed a series of studies and interventions focusing on bisexual men and their female partners which placed heavy emphasis on condom promotion and AIDS prevention within the broader context of reproductive health. More recently, since 1993, with support from both the USAID/Family Health International AIDSCAP Project and the Brazilian Ministry of Health, the Brazilian Interdisciplinary AIDS Association (ABIA) has coordinated a large-scale intervention project directed to men who have sex with men in general, which has combined outreach work, risk counselling and educational materials aimed at eroticizing safer sexual practices, on the one hand, with various forms of cultural activism aimed at responding to sexual stigma and discrimination. While none of these activities can hope to reach all men involved in homosexual and bisexual interactions, the gradual development of a range of social and psychological support services designed for men who have sex with men has been an important development which may offer a number of insights for the future.

On the basis of the work that has begun to be carried out, however, a range of different research and prevention activities can still be identified as key priorities in order to more effectively understand and respond to the role of bisexual behaviour in relation to HIV/AIDS in Brazil. First, there is an urgent need for further research aimed at documenting, through both qualitative and quantitative methods, the extent and patterning of bisexual behaviour. Random probability samples focusing on bisexual practices would obviously be of great interest, but are largely impractical, particularly given their relative lack of reliability in assessing stigmatized behaviours. As an alternative, more extensive targeted samples might be given priority, and attempts should be made to broaden the strategies for sampling and recruitment of subjects as much as possible.

While network or snowball sampling may continue to be a useful strategy for the study of bisexual behaviour, particularly if bisexuality itself is taken as the key characteristic used to construct the sample, every attempt should also be made to develop more extensive targeted recruiting outside such networks. Targeted recruiting in locations that serve as a focus for same-sex interactions should be a special priority, as these locations arguably serve as the most intensive available points of concentration for the populations under study. The use of ethnographic observation along with the application of a standardized interview schedule should make possible an assessment of the percentage of behaviourally homosexual as well as bisexual men frequenting different locations, as well as at least some indication of the levels of behavioural risk characterizing the different groups present in any given site. Ultimately, such data would be more useful, at least from the point of view of developing focused or targeted intervention activities, than the kinds of information collected through other possible research strategies.

In seeking to move from research to intervention, a number of related directions can also be recommended. While it is exceptionally difficult to identify the key issues that may be responsible for continued practice of high-risk behaviours, particularly on the basis of the relatively limited behavioural data that is currently available, it is nonetheless likely that not only attitudes towards risk itself, but also attitudes towards the desirability of condom use and the erotic satisfaction of different sexual acts are important factors. The social and cultural background, and the association made in popular culture between AIDS and homosexuality, may make many non-self-identified bisexual men unaware of their own risks, as well as less sensitive to the risks involved in relations with their female partners, and may even result in a process of denial in which confronting one's own risk would be tantamount to acknowledging carefully unacknowledged homosexual behaviours.

All of these factors, together with the persistent hidden or clandestine nature of so much bisexual behaviour, clearly suggests that outreach activities, risk assessment counselling, and social support structures may be as important as or more important than information alone in seeking to reach bisexual men and stimulate behavioural change. With the exception of a number of the outreach programmes described above, AIDS prevention activities developed thus far in Brazil have often placed greater emphasis on the development of educational materials than on the establishment of social support structures, and more interpersonal interventions, or interventions aimed at mobilizing community participation and political activism, have generally been lacking. Yet it is precisely interpersonal interaction and community mobilization that may be essential in building a bridge between the social/ sexual isolation that many bisexual men experience and the kinds of support that are necessary for risk-reducing behavioural change (Parker and Carballo, 1991).

The challenge of responding to the risk of HIV transmission in relation to bisexuality in Brazil is clearly complicated, and the activities that must be developed in order to meet this challenge are multiple. Further research aimed at documenting patterns of bisexual behaviour, assessing empirical levels of risk, and identifying possible strategies for risk reduction should be carried out as soon as possible. At the same time, the elaboration of strategies and techniques for outreach work and counselling should also move forward, and the evaluation of intervention strategies should be an integral part of AIDS prevention activities. The work that has already been carried out provides an important foundation for the work that must still be done. But the rapid spread of the HIV/AIDS epidemic in Brazil, and the on-going shift from predominantly homosexual to heterosexual transmission, suggest that the question of AIDS prevention in relation to bisexuality must be seen as increasingly central to both research and intervention agendas in the future.

### References

CASTILHO, E. *et al.* (1989) 'Patterns and Trends of Heterosexual Transmission of HIV among Brazilian AIDS Cases', paper presented at the Vth International Conference on AIDS, Montreal, Canada, Abstract M.G.P. 1.

CÔRTES, E. *et al.* (1989) 'Seroprevalence of HIV-1, HIV-2, and HTLV-I in

Brazilian Bisexual Males', paper presented at the Vth International Conference on AIDS, Montreal, Canada, Abstract M.G.P. 14.

DANIEL, H. and PARKER, R. (1991) *AIDS: A Terceira Epidemia*, São Paulo, Brasil, Iglu Editora.

DANIEL, H. and PARKER, R. (1993) *Sexuality, Politics and AIDS in Brazil*, London, Taylor & Francis.

FRY, P. (1982) *Para Inglês Ver: Identidade e Política na Cultura Brasileira*, Rio de Janeiro, Zahar.

FRY, P. (1985) 'Male Homosexuality and Spirit Possession in Brazil', *Journal of Homosexuality*, 11, pp. 137–53.

GUIMARÃES, C. D. (1994) 'Mulheres, Homens e AIDS: O Visível e o Invisível', in PARKER, R. *et al.* (Eds) *A AIDS no Brasil (1982–1992)*, Rio de Janeiro, Editora Relume-Dumará.

PARKER, R. G. (1985) 'Masculinity, Femininity, and Homosexuality: On the Anthropological Interpretation of Sexual Meanings in Brazil', *Journal of Homosexuality*, 11, pp. 155–63.

PARKER, R. G. (1987) 'Acquired Immunodeficiency Syndrome in Urban Brazil', *Medical Anthropology Quarterly*, New Series, 1, pp. 155–75.

PARKER, R. G. (1988) 'Sexual Culture and AIDS Education in Urban Brazil', in KULSTAD, R. (Ed.) *AIDS 1988: AAAS Symposia Papers*, Washington, DC, The American Association for the Advancement of Science.

PARKER, R. G. (1989) 'Youth, Identity, and Homosexuality: The Changing Shape of Sexual Life in Brazil', *Journal of Homosexuality*, 17, pp. 267–87.

PARKER, R. G. (1990) 'Responding to AIDS in Brazil', in MISZTEL, B. and MOSS, D. (Eds) *Action on AIDS: National Policies in Comparative Perspective*, Westport, CT, Greenwood Press.

PARKER, R. G. (1991) *Bodies, Pleasures, and Passions: Sexual Culture in Contemporary Brazil*, Boston, Beacon Press.

PARKER, R. G. (1994) *A Construção da Solidariedade: AIDS, Sexualidade e Política no Brasil*, Rio de Janeiro, Editora Relume-Dumará.

PARKER, R. G. and CARBALLO, M. (1990) 'Qualitative Research on Homosexual and Bisexual Behavior Relevant to HIV/AIDS', *Journal of Sex Research*, 27, pp. 497–525.

PARKER, R. G. and CARBALLO, M. (1991) 'Bisexual Behavior, HIV Transmission, and Reproductive Health', in CHEN, L. and SEPULVEDA, J. (Eds) *AIDS and Reproductive Health*, New York, Plenum Press.

PARKER, R. G. and TAWIL, O. (1991) 'Bisexual Behavior and HIV Transmission in Latin America', in TIELMAN, R., CARBALLO, M. and HENDRIKS, A. (Eds) *Bisexuality and HIV/AIDS: A Global Perspective*, New York, Prometheus.

PARKER, R. G., HERDT, G. and CARBALLO, M. (1991a) 'Sexual Culture, HIV Transmission, and AIDS Research', *Journal of Sex Research*, 28, pp. 77–98.

PARKER, R. G. *et al.* (1991b) 'Sexual Behavior and AIDS Awareness among Homosexual and Bisexual Men in Rio de Janeiro, Brazil', paper presented at the VIIth International Conference on AIDS, Florence, Italy.

PARKER, R. *et al.* (Eds) (1994) *A AIDS no Brasil (1982–1992)*, Rio de Janeiro, Editora Relume-Dumará.

RODRIGUES, L. and CHEQUER, P. (1989) 'AIDS in Brazil', *PAHO Bulletin*, 23, pp. 30–4.

SION, F. *et al.* (1989) 'Anal Intercourse: A Risk Factor for HIV Infection in Female Partners of Bisexual Men, Rio de Janeiro, Brazil', paper presented at the Vth International Conference on AIDS, Montreal, Canada, Abstract T.A.P. 117.

TURNER, C. F., MILLER, H. G. and MOSES, L. E. (Eds) (1989) *AIDS, Sexual Behavior, and Intravenous Drug Use*, Washington, DC, National Academy Press.

# Chapter 10

## Under the Blanket: Bisexualities and AIDS in India

*Shivananda Khan*

Contemporary debate about gender, sexuality, sexual behaviour and sexual health, and the implications of this debate for the development of appropriate and effective HIV prevention programmes, have become issues of great urgency for India. For if we do not have a sound appreciation of the central issues in this debate, if we cannot clearly define the parameters of what we mean by the term sexuality, and if we do not fully understand the cultural frameworks within which sexual behaviour occurs, we will not be able to develop effective interventions to decrease present rates of infection.

India already has an HIV/AIDS epidemic, but the ability of the Indian government to cope with the health care needs of people living with AIDS is seriously compromised by the strains placed upon the health delivery systems that currently exist. Primary, secondary and tertiary care are stretched beyond their capacity because of funding shortages, competing priorities, denial and the apparent 'invisibility' of AIDS. Such problems are compounded by fear, sexism, sex phobia, homophobia, and ignorance.

The World Health Organization estimates that between 1.5 million and 2 million people are currently living with HIV in India. Within the next decade, this figure may reach up to 20 million. The Harvard AIDS Institute's estimates are even higher, some 45 million infections (Mann *et al.*, 1992). South Asia has the fastest rate of increase of HIV infection in the world, and by 2020, if not before, will have more people living with HIV/AIDS than the combined number of cases in the rest of the world. Moreover, since AIDS-defining diseases develop earlier among people with HIV infection in India than in the West, by the end of the century, some one million people will be dying from AIDS.

In order to develop appropriate prevention strategies, we need to understand the dynamics of sexuality, the construction of gender, the psycho-social-cultural frameworks of sexual behaviour, and the contexts in which they exist in India. Unfortunately, all too often in the development of HIV prevention and outreach programmes, sexuality, identities, and sexual behaviours have been conceptualized within Eurocentric understandings and constructions.

In India, the main route of transmission has been reported as being unprotected penetrative sex. While recent estimates suggest that 70 per cent of all cases of transmission have occurred through heterosexual intercourse, this can be questioned, not only in terms of the actual figures, but in terms of the terminology used. Within the context of Indian cultures, heterosexual and homosexual identity-based frameworks do not exist in the sense in which they are understood in the West, and labelling behaviour as either heterosexual or homosexual does not explain what is happening sexually in India today.

Instead, and for many men at least, sexual experience and behaviour is more fluid. This is a consequence of many factors including gender segregation, Indian homosociability, the male ownership of public space, cultures of shame, community *izzat*,[1] the existence of compulsory and arranged marriages, the influence of joint and extended families, the lack of personal identity (or at the least the subsuming of this within family/community identity), and male and female roles as definers of adulthood. All of these factors have powerful effects on the construction and gendering of sexual behaviour.

### Male Bisexualities

While the emphasis in this chapter will be on male 'bisexualities' in India, this should in no way be taken as implying that Indian women are not sexually active either before or after marriage, that they are not particularly vulnerable to HIV and AIDS, or that they lack agency in relation to sexual and reproductive health. Rather, it is to suggest that an adequate understanding of vulnerability to infection should proceed from an appreciation of sexual life as it is lived, rather than as it is constructed for the individual through the categories of Western epidemiology, sexology and sexual politics.

Given the space available, what follows is a somewhat simplified, generalized and iconoclastic picture of sexual life, to which there will always be exceptions. But, as in the adage, exceptions prove the general rule. The analysis has derived from seven years' work in the fields of sexuality, sexual behaviour and HIV/AIDS within a South Asian context. Very little systematic research has been conducted in India into the nature of sexual behaviour, particularly amongst men who have sex with men. Most studies have been carried out within a broadly Eurocentric tradition, employing questionnaires and interview schedules that offer ready-made, and frequently culturally imposed descriptions of sexual behaviour as response options (e.g. heterosexual/homosexual). In consequence, people have not been encouraged to speak for themselves, except in very limited ways (Mane, 1992).

### Language

The human mind cannot think a thought unless the words to express the thought exist. (George Orwell, *1949*)

Language is essentially a cultural artefact. While languages are learned, they are not acquired in a vacuum. The process of learning takes place within the context of interacting perceptions, beliefs, experiences of the past and present, and expectations of the future. And words themselves carry a socially constructed history of their own. All these mediate and condition both the learning of language, and the meanings with which words are imbued. This has enormous implications for the communication of thoughts and ideas, as well as for the sharing of information. More specifically, in relation to sexual health, HIV/AIDS and sexual behaviour, how do we ensure the development of a shared understanding of the issues we are speaking about? Most cultures have constructed taboos around sexual behaviours, particularly those that are not seen as socially and/or religiously acceptable, or that are defined as 'abnormal', 'sinful', 'evil' – words that can carry strong emotions of guilt, shame, dishonour and fear. In many cultures, sex lies within the invisible realm, and very often there are no commonly available appropriate terms to discuss sex and sexual behaviours in the public arena.

Different cultures place differing values on the various sexual aspects of our lives. These values are often concealed within the words used by these cultures to describe and/or name these sexual aspects. Direct correlations between the words used in one language and those used in another do not always exist. Translations between one language and another can carry enormous risks of misinformation, misunderstanding and downright censorship.

With the medicalization of sexuality and sexual behaviour in Western cultures since the nineteenth century, a whole new language has evolved to describe sexual behaviours. More specifically, a naming process developed which categorized and labelled peoples by their sexual practices, creating the terms homosexual, heterosexual, bisexual and so on, along with the personality traits and social characteristics that were assumed to apply to such labelled persons (Foucault, 1987; Weeks, 1991). A person expressing same-sex behaviours thereby became *a* homosexual, a new construction. Procreative heterosexuality became the normative process. The dichotomized, oppositional, and hierarchical structures of male and female also framed homosexuality and heterosexuality. One was either masculine or feminine, heterosexual or homosexual (despite the special category of bisexual). The concomitant discourse of sexuality that came into being carried its own seeds of self-definition and was to some extent tautological. Within all this, the heterosexual was sexually defined as *only* having vaginal sex, whilst the homosexual was defined as *only* having anal sex. For a man to have anal sex with a woman was often not considered, being an invisible behaviour.

The word homosexual, as it is understood in the West, does not have a direct equivalent in Indian community languages. This does not imply that 'homosexual' behaviours do not exist. What it means is that these behaviours have different histories, different contexts and different constructions, and are thus named differently. For example, the act of penetration is a definer of phallic power, a male signifier. For a person to be penetrated is to define that person as 'not a man'. The language of male penetration is around gender and power. So *gandu* and *khusra*[2] are words sometimes used synonymously with the term homosexual, but they are not the same. They represent men who are penetrated, and have meanings to do with a lack of masculinity and malehood, describing a person who is 'not a man' and 'not a woman', but of a third gender. In a similar way, the term *hijra*[3] means a person of a third gender.

While these terms are abusive, derogatory and degrading, we need to be careful in analysing their meaning. For in India, malehood and femalehood are also defined as family, community and social duties. A man can be extremely 'effeminate' in his behaviour (in the way in which the term is defined in the West), but because he fulfils his community duties as a married man with sons, he is defined as manly, a proper man. Furthermore, a boy (who is male but not yet a man in terms of social duties and responsibilities) may be extremely masculine (in a Western sense), but is still defined as not-yet-a-man. He is, after all, not married with sons. This establishes the framework for specific gender constructions around post-pubescent boys who are not yet 'men', and who constitute the 'beardless youths' of Arab and Mughul Indian sexual histories.[4]

### Culture

But language alone is insufficient to explain how sexual life is lived. How we conduct ourselves and how our lives are constructed, how actions are given meaning and content, what value systems we abide by and the worldview that we have are some of the elements that constitute the dominant meanings within a culture. Culture here is taken to mean the wholeness of a particular community, the social values, contexts of family, religion, marriage, personal relationships, lifestyles, language, traditions and customs. Three aspects of culture are of key importance to an understanding of men's sexuality in India today: the family, marriage and religion. Each will be examined separately, before interconnections between them are explored.

#### Family

Within Indian communities, there are extremely strong links within the family. Here, the family is much more than the immediate biological parents and siblings. It includes all the relatives – grand-parents and their relatives, uncles and aunts, brothers-in-law and sisters-in law, nephews and nieces, and even distant cousins. The Indian family is a joint and extended family, constituting a community in its own right, defined by language, dialect, religious practice, caste, place of origin, and so on. Often whole villages are made of interconnected families.

These links are held together by custom, tradition, belief, practice and economics. Their value lies in providing a form of social security and welfare in a culture that has neither. The elders are supported, as are the unemployed, the unmarried, children and the disabled. It is considered a moral duty for the family to stay together in this mutual support system, whether such staying together is physical or psychological.

Such extended family systems can be liberating in relation to the social conditions of individual members. To rely on the family for support – be it emotional, physical, or financial – relieves much of the burden for sustaining the self. But in consequence, individuality can become lost. There is no space for it, with personal choice and desire becoming subsumed within family choice and desire. The person is replaced by the family. In this context there can be little space for personal identity as a central means of self-definition. Who you are individually is of less importance than which family you are a part of (Kakar, 1989).

This means that in India people tend to stay much longer within the family household than do their European counterparts. There are a significant number of men and women over 30, for example, who still live with their parents, who are still single, and who are still considered and treated as children, not as adults (Kakar, 1989). Such single people are often not single by choice, however. The economics of marriage have begun to affect when it takes place. Particularly in urban areas, the need to find a home, dowry, and the cost of living have all delayed marriage to later and later ages. Many men are now marrying in their late twenties or thirties (Khan, 1990, 1994).

At the same time, the social demand for sons as primary income generators has meant that the life expectancy for female children is much lower than that for males. In India, 1991 census data indicate there are 928 women for every 1,000 men. This means that there is a significant and growing shortage of women for men to marry. Or to put it another way, there is a surplus of sexually active men.

For the vast majority of people living with their parents there is no personal space. One-room or two-room households, holding parents and several siblings, are common. Within these households, there will be a male space and a female space for sleeping. Such cramped 'male space' in a culture with high levels of homosociability establishes fertile conditions for *maasti*[5] and the release of 'bodily tensions'. These quick and often furtive sexual gropings occur as invisible behaviours – being behaviours of the dark, behaviours 'under the blanket' – and therefore are not 'real'.

In India, you *never* leave the family home. You carry the psychological space within you all the time. When crowded living conditions generate intense arguments, disagreements and family fights, all members of the extended family, and sometimes even the neighbours, may join in, usually on the side of parents. This is reinforced by the belief that it is the *duty* of the child to obey the parent, whatever the age of the child. Obedience to parental demands and pressures is one of the central glues that is perceived as holding the family together. To disobey one's parents is to bring shame and dishonour upon the family.

Parents are responsible for their children. In Indian cultures, adulthood and adult responsibilities are conferred *after* marriage and, for a woman, after her first-born son. These become the 'rites of passage'. Personal privacy as a concept and a right is not embedded within Indian cultures. What is private is the family, and depending on the particular issue or context, this could mean the immediate biological family, the extended family or the community as a whole. This form of privacy is not shaped by a recognition of need for such privacy. Rather it is motivated by traditional concepts of *honour* and *shame.* Honour here is not so much that which is deemed honourable as it is a community perception. Shame is not so much that which may be deemed as wrongful (or even sinful), but conduct that brings shame to the family and/or community as a whole. These two intersecting frameworks arise out of understandings of value systems around what is *public* and what is *private.*

For the family, honour is therefore a possession, not a quality. Shame is an expression of honour being lost. Both of these elements are public events. Public behaviour, behaviour that is visible, is bound within a sense of community duty, honour and obligation. In such a context any behaviour which is visible to the community falls within the scope of public behaviour and therefore falls within the boundaries of honour and shame. If the behaviour is not *visible*, then it does not exist. Through such invisibility, honour in the community is maintained, there is no shame, and all remains well.

Such systems of public and private can lead to denial of what are deemed socially unacceptable behaviours, because of their relative invisibility in the public domain. Claims are often made that such behaviours 'do not exist within our communities', or that they are 'not part of our culture'. Evidence which contradicts such a view is frequently dismissed as the effects of Western culture.[6] When an individual behaves in ways deemed to bring dishonour or shame to the family, extended family and/or community, the reaction can often be severe – exile, excommunication, physical abuse, and sometimes death. Or there will be emotional or financial blackmail by family members to force conformity to family dictates.

Events that occur in a public space may not be considered public if they are not observed, or, if observed, not discussed. For example, in a public toilet in Calcutta where male-to-male sexual activity takes place every evening, there are no lights. With no public lighting, such a setting becomes a private space. The inside of the toilet is visible from the street because of the street lighting and at times individuals will stop and look into the toilet, often seeing two men involved in a sexual act in the semi-dark. But this is still a private event because there is no discussion by the observer. It only becomes a public event that can then bring shame when there is open discussion, the police arrive, or the observer makes loud comments.[7]

Marriage

Marriage is *the* central issue within people's lives, where it is the mainstay of family and/or community life. It can be seen as a compulsory duty towards maintaining family and community ties, and it is part of the definition of manhood and femalehood. Not to be married means you are not an adult. The exception is that of the *sadhu*[8] or *bramacharaya*, the person who sacrifices duty and family in search of god as a 'sexless' being, an ascetic who has sacrificed their sense of malehood or femalehood for a higher cause. This does not mean, of course, that all *sadhus* do not have sex. There are some who have sex with their *chelas*,[9] or with others, both women and men. In Hindu traditions, spiritual sanctity can carry great sexual potency, while Tantric traditions often have a strong sexual component.

Traditionally, marriages are arranged between two extended families, and such arrangements are based on economic and inter-family connections. Nowadays, amongst middle-class and upper-class families, parents may ask their children about the suitability of their choices, and there are processes whereby the two prospective partners can meet each other regularly before a wedding. Very often such meetings are chaperoned by some parental figure. While such choice may be significant, ultimately there is no choice about marriage itself. For the majority of women and men, individual choice is subsumed within family choice.

Where there is resistance from a son or daughter towards marriage, enormous pressure can be brought to bear to submit to the parent's/family's wishes. As the child gets older, such pressures increase and some families will use emotional blackmail, financial inducements, threats, excommunication, and sometimes violence to enforce the family dictates. To remain unmarried can be seen as an aberration, a sickness, bringing shame and dishonour upon the family. Something must be wrong with the person and/or with the family. The family could not find a marriage partner, or the child has a problem, or they could not afford the dowry, and so on. The pressures on young women are particularly intense. At least the young man can use a greater range of excuses – business commitments, education, travel, etc.

Marriage is not seen as an option for choice. It is seen as an essential requirement of maintaining the family, as a family duty, as a sign of obedience to parents. Rather than resist and challenge parental wishes, Indian men and women will often get married to the choice of their parents. As a room service man interviewed in Bombay during 1992 as part of an on-going study of sexual behaviour put it:

> I didn't want to get married. But what can I do? My parents pushed and pushed. Every day my mother would nag me, my father would nag me. They would invite other families to the house so I could 'view' the daughters. I finally just gave in. And when I finally said yes, my parents were so happy. But what about me?

Few married men inform their wives about their extra-marital behaviour. In the main, many believe that all they need to do to function adequately as husbands is offer economic support to their wives and engage in sexual intercourse in order to have children. There are many men who will only have sexual intercourse with their wives a few times a year specifically to get their wives pregnant (Kakar, 1989). Often there is no joy in such intercourse. It is seen as a duty – duty as an adult male, duty to the wife and family, and as part of the duty to have children. As one person in a recent sexual health workshop in Orissa put it, 'I do duty to my wife'.

The wife, sometimes seen as an Honoured Partner, cannot be touched by sexual desire, thereby assuming the role of mother, sister, or bearer of the husband's children. Such desires are part of another construction. Sex for procreation is what occurs in marriage. Sex for pleasure is what occurs outside the marriage. It is considered natural for men to be 'lustful'. Sex for pleasure and sex as lust are often seen as synonymous. This leads to significant numbers of married men having sex outside their marriage. And as long as this behaviour is invisible, it brings no shame and dishonour to the family. Public life is separated from private life. And if women are not accessible or cannot be afforded, then other men or young boys are more so. It is not so much a matter of sexual desire as sexual discharge. As one man interviewed in New Delhi in 1992 described it:

> Yeah, I have sex with my wife, perhaps once a month. I don't enjoy it. I rather not do it. But I have to keep her satisfied. She's complained about it to me, but I just shrug my shoulders, you know, pretend that I don't really like sex. It's all very, what's the word? Perfunctory, you know, get on, get off sort of thing. What can I do? I do go out to find men with whom I can have sex.

What we have here is a cultural framework of compulsory penetrative and procreative sexual intercourse. Other forms of sexual activity not connected to procreation are for pleasure, but very often the only route to express these sexual behaviours is outside the marriage – hidden, invisible and under the blanket. Such a patterning of sexual behaviour has major implications for the practice of safer sex, for to use condoms with one's wife creates two tensions. First, it does not enable the couple to fulfil the central requirement of the marriage – children. Second, using a condom generates suspicion. Because of this women find themselves very vulnerable. They carry responsibility for family honour and tradition, and whenever issues arise that question this honour, it is the woman who is victimized.

A married woman's options may be severely limited. Not only her own family, but members of her husband's family will place enormous pressure to maintain a marriage. Divorce rates in India are still relatively low, not because marriages work better than in the West, but because divorce and separation carry dishonour and shame for both families. The public perception of a marriage that maintains itself must be upheld.

Even where men who have sex with other men have acquired some sort of 'gay sensibility' in the Western sense, this too becomes restricted, buried under the weight of tradition and custom. As a gay-identified man interviewed in New Delhi in 1992 explained:

> I can't tell my wife about myself. It would destroy my family and her. I can't have a divorce because of the effect it would have on my family as well as her. What would happen to her? I go out several times a month, pick up some guy and stay the night at some local cheap hotel. Or maybe drop by the cruising place on my way home from work in the evening. The wife always has a go at me when I am late home, or stay out the night. I have to really think on the excuses I make. But what can I do? I got married because my family wanted me to. They chose her for me. I just said yes.

### Religion

The main religions of India are Hinduism, Islam and Sikhism and to some extent Indian Christianity. It is not appropriate here to discuss each of these religions in terms of their specific and particular beliefs, traditions, and practices. What it is more important to explore is the interaction between religion, culture and social dynamics. For example, Bengali Muslims, while having the same faith as Pakistani Muslims, will often have very different customs and traditions. This is because of different languages, different histories, different geographies, etc. Furthermore, while sometimes these religions may be seen as monolithic, they are not. Islam, for example, has several different denominations. Each follows the Koran and the Hadith, but each has its own traditions and customs, based upon a specific interpretation of the Hadith and the Koran, be they Sunni, Shia, Sufi, Ishmaili or whatever. Similarly Hinduism is not constructed around a central person, creed or doctrine, but is a broad and eclectic system of beliefs and doctrines. Sikhism arose from an attempt to unify the beliefs of Islam and Hinduism. Of course, this is oversimplistic. These faiths are much more complicated than this, with historical traditions that through accretion over time have often added their own cultural nuances.

What needs to be emphasized is that religion and culture are not isolated from each other, nor do they represent the same thing; rather, they are held together via complex dynamics. While religions specify particular social practices, beliefs and attitudes, very often cultural traditions and customs will outweigh religious beliefs and statements. What matters is interpretation of the latter, and who does it. Where an interpretation of religious texts interpenetrates with dominant cultural beliefs and customs, very often these customs and practices take on a sanctity that never existed before.

It should also be remembered that in contrast to the way that Christianity is practised in the West, where personal choice is emphasized, the religions of India relate more closely to how communities function as a whole. Religious and secular life centres in the mosque, the temple and the *gurdwara*.[10] Public faith in a specific system of beliefs, whether Hindu, Islam or Sikh, is not separated from the day-to-day life of the person, but is an integral part of community and public life.

This does not mean that there is not intense personal belief and practice. Of course there is. There is the private *namaz*,[11] the personal prayer, the *puja*[12] at home. For many, religion provides personal solace and meaning to life. But with all this go the daily observances, the food a person eats, his or her relationships with the family, interactions with the community, religious celebrations and festivals: all are interlinked and interdependent. This is the visible side, the proof of one's religious observance. Private and public are co-joined, which means that there will be those for whom only the public observance matters, those whose private practice may not be in line with public observance. It is wrong to see this as 'hypocrisy' though, because the public and private spheres have different meanings from those of the West.

What this means is that public belief and private practice can be at variance without creating undue social or personal dissonance. A person can be a practising Muslim or Hindu or Sikh, obeying all the social rules that these faiths require, but as long as the sexual behaviour remains invisible, to some extent it does not exist. And within all of these faiths, marriage and procreative sex is compulsory. A man is either married or going to be married. Within such frameworks, shame, gender segregation and virginity become contexts creating social spaces for an increased incidence of sex between men. One can practise these behaviours without causing shame or stigma because of their invisibility.

### Romance and Friendship

What has love got to do with marriage? This is a question often voiced in India. The dominant expectation and hope is that love will grow after the marriage, but for not insignificant numbers of women and men, this only remains an illusion. India is filled with romance. It is always visible, always present. In any of the ubiquitous Hollywood films, the hero and the heroine sing romantic and chaste love songs to each other. They go through the trials and tribulations that the three hours demand, and if their families will agree to the match, they can get married and sexual fulfilment will follow. The key to all of this is the families' agreement. For if such romance cuts across race, caste, sub-caste, religion or economic group, the likelihood is that such romantic dreams cannot be fulfilled, with the death of one of the partners being a not uncommon outcome. The family always wins in so far as marriage is concerned.

In terms of Indian cultural norms, direct relationships between men and women before marriage, be they social or sexual, are frowned upon and socially unacceptable. Such socialization is seen as allowing the possibility of dishonouring the woman's family. Men are seen as naturally lustful, uncontrollable, while young women are seen as being able to arouse that lust. Women must therefore be protected from men's lust, while men must be protected from 'women's wiles'. In this sense, the public domain is owned by males. For a woman to be seen with a man who is not a relative or husband can result in damaging and dishonouring gossip. Families therefore police their young women. To be seen out in the evening on your own as a woman is to risk being given the label 'evening person' or prostitute. To kiss a woman who is not married to you, or to hold her hand in public, is to risk dishonouring her, and in some cases the man will also risk abuse and violence. Displays of physical affection for a woman must occur behind closed doors. But what if such privacy is not available? For many young men, women are simply not accessible. Romantic longings are therefore unfulfilled. For many men, sex workers are the only women available, but here love only rarely enters the equation, and for many men the financial costs are high.

For many men across all ages, emotional and sexual energy, romantic longing and affectional needs tend to be channelled between themselves. Intense friendships are formed within homoaffectionalist frameworks that include extensive male-to-male touching, the holding of hands, close body contact and sleeping together in crowded spaces. This should not be taken as implying that all men in India are having sex with each other. India, as a homosocial culture in which women are difficult for men to access either for friendship or for sex, has created social spaces where it is acceptable, if not encouraged, for men to show affection to each other, both publicly and in private. But the line between homoaffectionalism in such a supportive environment and actual homosexual behaviour is very fine, and many men are likely to cross it in contexts that allow the behaviour to remain invisible (Hardman, 1993; Khan, 1994).

An illustration of this is provided by an event that occurred while visiting a single-room home in New Delhi shared by the parents, four children, one a male in his mid-teens, and an uncle of the children. The male teenager and the uncle were sharing a blanket while the female members of the household were getting on with the housekeeping. After a while it became clear what the two males were doing under the blanket, a behaviour totally ignored by the women. Subsequent discussion with the uncle revealed that during the night the two young men would often masturbate together under their shared blanket, and on some occasions, the older would penetrate the younger when everyone was asleep. Because the behaviour was invisible, there did not appear to be any sense of shame or guilt. As the uncle put it, 'What can I do? I get body tension. He gets body tension. We are together. It just happens. We are friends.' When asked will he get married, this same man replies 'Of course'. When asked would he have sex with a woman if he had the opportunity, he replies 'Of course'. When asked has he had sex with other men, he replies 'Of course' under similar circumstances!

What identity is operating here? Who is the heterosexual or the homosexual, and who the bisexual? Terminology becomes inadequate, for it reduces the complexity of desire and discharge into a nominal framework whereas, as this example illustrates, sexual behaviour here is fluid, contextualized by space, time and opportunity. Existing labels imply a fixity to sexual desire and behaviour. These are not relevant in the Indian context described here.

This behaviour is closely linked to understandings of sexual behaviour in Indian cultures and is contextualized within a concept which in Hindi is called *maasti.* The word is not easily translated, but can be defined as mischief – mischief in a playful sense, and with strong sexual connotations, usually between unmarried men, youths and boys and between friends. It is not seen as a serious act, because it does not involve a woman, nor is it seen as sex very often. To some extent this sexual play is even socially permissible – 'young men letting of steam' – so long as it remains invisible. The invisibility of *maasti* does not differentiate this form of sexual playfulness from others, for all sexual behaviour, whether socially legitimate or not, must also remain invisible. But in the context of *maasti*, there is a form of social legitimation of sex between friends, not publicly spoken about, but accepted.

Despite the existence of intense friendships that produce visible physical affection between males of all ages, that sometimes lead to sexual acts between friends (and if there is an age difference between the two males, the older one may penetrate the younger), and that might in other circumstances be described as 'gay', such an identity does not exist for the persons concerned. Sex with another man is not so much a permanent feature as an additional outlet. The expectation is that one day the same person will be married and have children, and perhaps then able to afford sex with a female prostitute. Within this context, sexual behaviour is not so much an expression of personal identity as a behaviour linked to opportunity, accessibility and the desire for sexual discharge. This should not be taken as implying, however, that loving bonds between men do not exist. They do, but they are bounded by the cultural necessity of marriage and children.

Beyond the situations described, there exist specialized contexts in which men can seek out other men for sex. Since there are no 'gay' bars, clubs or discotheques, these are most usually public spaces such as the street, the bus stand, the park, the public toilet, the railway or bus station. Such publicness leads to quick sex, penetrative or otherwise, in the darkness of parks and toilets, behind bushes, in alleyways and on beaches. Passing workers may join in the networks. Whether this is for sexual release, money, or the desire to have sex with other men is a difficult question to answer. Taxi-drivers, rickshaw wallahs, *mallaish wallahs*,[13] room service boys and housekeeping men in hotels, waiters at restaurants, shop assistants, the framework is ubiquitous. The glance, the second glance, the smile, the appropriate questions, sometimes 'for a few rupees more', sometimes just *maasti*. In Indian urban cultures, male-to-male sex does not take place only in a few selected areas as in Western cities. It can occur anywhere, in the right conditions, at the right time, and in the right space.

For the middle classes, domestic servants may be sexually available too, be they male or female. There is evidence to suggest that sex between the young male sons and the young (and sometimes not so young male) servants may not be as rare as is popularly believed. Such behaviour is not simply an urban phenomenon. Discussions over the years with several hundred village men between the ages of 15 and 30 suggest that sex between men also occurs in village environments – in the fields, in the dark, and in the home under 'shared blankets'. Much of this sex may be between relatives: uncles and nephews, cousins, in-laws, where there is space and time.

What this suggests is that in India, sexual behaviour between males may be common but hidden. It is invisible, not only because it is outside the public gaze, but also because no one talks about it. But within this context, the behaviour is bound within the necessity for marriage, desire for opportunistic sex with women, access to sexual space and so on. Further, the definitions that exist regarding male-to-male sex, terms such as '*hijra*' or 'homosexual', act as frames hiding such levels of activity.

What is the best terminology to use to describe the patterns of behaviour that have been described? Are they the bisexualities that the title of this book implies, or are they something different? And what are the implications of such patterns of behaviour for HIV prevention? These are issues that will be addressed in the final section of this chapter.

### The Challenge for HIV Prevention

Earlier it was suggested that the HIV epidemic may be reaching crisis proportions in India, and that much of the cause of this crisis stems from a refusal to face the reality of Indian sexual behaviours, of which a significant component is male-to-male sex within broader cultural dynamics that have a major impact upon both women and men. But there are a host of other factors that have serious impact on the ability to develop effective prevention programmes, as well as care and support for those already infected. These include poor sex education for young people, either at home or in schools, poor knowledge of condoms and how to use them, lack of time and space in which to have safer sex, and high reported rates of STDs which may increase the likelihood of HIV transmission. Moreover, in urban areas at least, high levels of environmental pollution, polluted water, adulterated food, poor hygienic conditions, corrupt officials, overcrowded public hospitals, expensive private hospitals, poor knowledge of HIV among the medical profession, ignorance about HIV transmission, and AIDS phobia mean that the time elapsing between infection and illness or death can be much shorter than in the West.

HIV-related prevention work in India still focuses primarily on target groups such as long-distance truck drivers, female sex workers and injecting drug users, and here much of what is done is inadequate. For example, work with injecting drug users tends to focus more on injection-related risks than on the possibility of sexual transmission. As yet, relatively little work has been undertaken to address the HIV/AIDS health promotion needs of men who have sex with other men, be they 'gay-identified', 'bisexual' or otherwise. At the time of writing, only three small projects in the whole of India received any sort of funding or support. The majority of more mainstream projects neglect the fact that men have sex with men as well as with women and that for significant numbers of unmarried men, sex with other men is their only outlet, be it driven by desire or opportunity. Still less is it acknowledged that men also have anal sex with women. By working from Eurocentric notions of sexual identity and by working within a heterosexual/homosexual framework, prevention efforts miss the majority of male-to-male sexual behaviours.

For many people, sexual behaviour takes the place of sexuality. Women's sexual behaviour becomes controlled and marginalized, if not denied. Male sexual behaviour becomes self-absorbed, being reduced to discharge rather than a desire for the other person. Sexual behaviour becomes depersonalized and brutalized, regardless of whether it occurs between male and female, or male and male. Concepts of personal choice and of privacy become lost, there being serious limits to the development of what elsewhere is understood as individuality. If we are to move towards forms of society that enable all people to express their best, that give people the opportunity to develop personhood, that enable people to make choices about their sexuality and sexual/emotional desires, that empower people to make positive decisions about their own sexual health and that of others, then it will be necessary to challenge the principles that define sexual life in these terms. There is however a small but growing movement amongst those whose sense of personal identities and emotional and sexual desires are outside the socially constructed 'norm', to create new forms of identities that enable them to express their desires in healthy and more caring ways. Many of these *may* well call themselves lesbians, gay men, bisexuals and even heterosexuals.

The impact of such developments is, however, extremely marginal on the vast majority of men who have sex with other men. Often non-educated and working-class, from urban and rural areas, their desires are shaped by other factors. In Hinduism and Islam, celibacy and abstinence are not central to dominant structures of belief. And although the idea circulates that sex should take place only within marriage, social and cultural arrangements more strongly facilitate sex between men than between men and women. It may be helpful, therefore, to see heterosexuality as part of a broader spectrum of alternate sexualities and their expression.

In relation to AIDS, it is essential to develop a full range of prevention strategies if there is not to be a huge personal, social, cultural and economic impact. There should be a public acknowledgment of the fact that men have sex with other men – not only as 'gay' men, but also as part of the sexual repertoire of large numbers of sexually active boys and men.

This can be approached in terms of two specific strategies. Firstly, in any discussion of sexual behaviours, in training, condom promotion, HIV/AIDS prevention campaigns, sex education, information resources, anal sex must feature prominently – both anal sex between men, and anal sex between men and women. There should be equal prominence given to this behaviour and and it should be featured alongside vaginal sex. This should be done through a safer-sex approach rather than in a condemnatory way. To stigmatize this behaviour even more is to increase its invisibility, making it more difficult to access its practitioners and even more difficult to promote safer sex behaviours. These issues should be discussed in high schools, colleges and universities, as well as in STD clinics, factories, bazaars, and as part of general campaigns. All this requires an increase in discussion about sexual behaviours, not within the context of 'heterosexual' or 'homosexual' identities but in the context of the behaviours themselves.

The second approach must parallel the above. It involves urgently beginning direct intervention and outreach work amongst men who have sex with men. The most effective method in such intervention strategies is to use people who already participate in such behaviours and who are part of existing sexual networks. Peer intervention strategies have always been seen as the most successful in enabling and empowering people to modify their sexual behaviours. Role modelling, mimicry, hero-worship and imitation are frameworks that have been used successfully in a variety of settings. But this also requires a process of empowerment to enable men who have sex with men to talk about their behaviours, the risks, and the responsibilities to each other and their families. It also means the creation of safe spaces where such discussions can take place.

Both strategies require the de-stigmatization of sex between men, and its decriminalization. They also call for extensive training of political, health and social staff and volunteers, the medical profession, and family planning staff. Finally, they require a commitment from the political and health leadership in the country. If we are too timid in our approaches, dealing only with 'gay' issues and with 'heterosexual' issues, we will fail to intervene around some of the most important ways in which HIV is transmitted in India today.

### Notes

1 *Izzat* is an Urdu term for honour.
2 *Gandu*, a Hindi term, is an abusive word roughly meaning a man who is not

a man, a man who is fucked, a man who is without testicles and deserves to be fucked. *Khusra*, an Urdu term, has similar connotations.

3 *Hijra* is a Hindi term.

4 The Hanbalite (Islamic school of jurisprudence) jurisconsult Ibn al Gauzi (died 1200) wrote: 'He who claims that he experiences no desire when looking at beautiful boys or youths is a liar, and if we could believe him, he would be an animal, not a human being.' Abu Nuwas (*c.* 810), a famous Arab poet, wrote:

> Jealous people and slanders overwhelm me with sarcasm
> because my lover has started to shave
> I answer them: friends, how wrong you are!
> Since when has fuzz been a flaw?
> It enhances the splendour of his lips and teeth,
> like silk cloth which is brightened by pearls.
> And I consider myself fortunate that his sprouting beard
> preserves his beauty from indiscreet glances;
> it gives his kisses a different flavour
> and makes a reflection glisten on the silver of his cheeks.

Of Sultan Mahood Mirza (uncle of Babur, founder of the Mughal Empire in India), it is written:

> He took beautiful boys of his noblemen and admitted them into his 'boys' harem'. He surrounded himself with scores of beautiful boys. This practice became a custom throughout his kingdom and noblemen occupied themselves with this mode. (Tuzk-I-Babur, autobiography of Babur, fifteenth century)

5 *Maasti* is a Hindi term meaning mischief.

6 Statements to this effect were made by Indian Government health officials at the International Conference on AIDS, Montreal, 1990. In 1994, the National Federation of Women West Bengal branch, on hearing of a conference for gay men and men who have sex with men in Bombay, called homosexuality 'a Western disease', and asked for the meeting to be banned.

7 This observation arose from a discussion with a local 'gay' group in Calcutta as well as a site visit.

8 A *sadhu* is a wandering Hindu ascetic. *Fakhir* is the Muslim version.

9 A *chela* is a student of a *guru* (teacher).

10 A *gurdwara* is a Sikh temple.

11 *Namaz* is a Muslim ritual prayer which according to the Koran should be offered five times a day. It consists of specific words and acts.

12 *Puja* is a Hindu act of worship and ritual offering to the family god or goddess.

13 *Mallaish wallahs* are boys/men who give massages.

### References

FOUCAULT, M. (1987) *The History of Sexuality, Volume 1*, Harmondsworth, Penguin Books.

HARDMAN, P. (1993) *Homoaffectionalism*, London, GLB Books.

KAKAR, S. (1989) *Intimate Relations and the Inner World*, Harmondsworth, Penguin Books.

KHAN, S. (1990) *The Khush Report*, London, Naz Project.

KHAN, S. (1994) *Contexts – Race, Culture and Sexuality*, London, Naz Project.

MANE, P. (1992) *AIDS Prevention: The Sociocultural Context in India*, Bombay, Tata Institute of Social Sciences.

MANN, J. *et al.* (1992) *AIDS in the World*, Boston, MA, Harvard University Press.

ORWELL, G. (1949) *1984*, London, Secter & Warburg.

WEEKS, J. (1991) *Against Nature: Essays on History, Sexuality and Identity*, London, Rivers Oram Press.

## Chapter 11

# Male Homosexual Behaviour and HIV-Related Risk in China

*Suiming Pan*
*with Peter Aggleton*

Before the revolution in 1949, China had a long history of male behavioural homosexuality within its rayal dynasties (Van Gulick, 1961; Ruan and Tsai, 1988; Lau and Ng, 1989; Hinsch, 1990). A tolerance for male sexual diversity can be found throughout Chinese history and is recorded in a well-developed literature. Such tolerance allowed men openly to show their sexual desires and orientation, particularly if the person concerned was literate, or of the court. The surviving literature demonstrates unequivocally an acceptance of homosexual behaviour among men by the royal courts, its practice being widespread among the nobility. Both the famous story of the *Long Yang* set in the Spring-Autumn and Warring States Period (770–221 BCE), and the story of the *Cut Down Sleeve* set in the Han dynasty (206 BCE–220 CE), contain accounts of courtly love between rulers and subjects, homosexuality being seen as a noble virtue (Hinsch, 1990). From the Yuan dynasty onwards (1279–1368), and with the growth of urban populations and the appearance of the novel, accounts of homosexual behaviour among the common people increased, reaching a peak in the late Ming dynasty (1368–1644), a representative work being *Bian Er Chai* which contains four stories of male homosexuality among the then middle class. Detailed descriptions of anal sex between men can be found in scores of other erotic novels, as can mention of male prostitution.

Some writers claim that the transformation of homosexuality into something negative is a relatively recent phenomenon, occurring in the Manchu-dominated Qin dynasty, during the final years of dynastic rule (Hinsch, 1990). While this is probably true, the reasons for such a transformation are more complex than is often suggested, and go beyond a reaction at the time to Ming permissiveness, and a desire to promote a neo-Confucian familism. Two main contributing factors can be distinguished (Pan, 1988). The first of these relates to the minority status of the Manchu rulers. Because of their numerical disadvantage, members of the Qin dynasty were required to exert their influence through the control of thoughts, ideas and popular feelings, rather than through direct military rule. Emperors from Kang-xi to Qian-long in the seventeenth and eighteenth centuries viewed folk customs and everyday social practices as the bedrock of popular sentiment. They therefore sought to control all erotic literary works, pictures and devices used for sexual pleasure. These interventions in the field of popular sexual practice marked a major change in the relationship between the aristocracy and the peasantry. Hitherto, a more informal policy of live and let live had prevailed. The interventions by the Manchu rulers rendered the overt expression of sexuality ideological and political, imbuing it with the negative connotations that persist today. Additionally, dominant sexual beliefs and ideologies during this period, especially those promoted by scholars of the so-called *li-xue* (a school of idealist philosophy that became popular after the Ming dynasty) reflected a mixture of Confucian, Taoist and Buddhist ideas, being far removed from earlier and purer Confucian teachings emphasizing the naturalness of human sexual expression.

Between 1840 and 1911, following greater contact with the West, a distinction came to be drawn between traditional practices and newer ideas. Traditional customs which had persisted for thousands of years, such as having concubines, visiting brothels, hiring another man's wife in order to have a son, and foot binding, disappeared with the advent of so-called modern society. Swept away with these traditional practices were traditional patterns of homosexual behaviour between men.

Though Mao Zedong and Jiang Jieshi were rivals in every other sense, on one thing they agreed: homosexuality harked back to some form of bad cultural heritage. Each vied with the other to prove that they were not only more advanced than the former dynasty, but also more forceful than the other in their rejection of homosexuality. Until the mid-1980s, behaviourally homosexual men were routinely imprisoned or placed in forced labour camps (Stafford, 1967; Butterfield, 1982; Ruan and Tsai, 1988; Ruan, 1991). Of one thousand behaviourally homosexual men surveyed in 1992, 8.2 per cent reported having received some kind of official punishment and a further 2.9 per cent had been blackmailed.

Change was not immediate following the death of Mao Zedong in 1976 and the beginning of reforms (Hinsch, 1990; Ruan, 1991). Even now the tendency to see the world idealistically rather than in terms of empirical reality leads the authorities to underplay the existence of homosexual behaviour among men (Gil, 1991, 1992). A recent article in *Qou Shi*, a prestigious communist party journal, stated that homosexuality, an 'ugly phenomenon typical only of the old society', had been wholly eradicated since the liberation in 1949.

Given the history described, it is somewhat paradoxical that male homosexuality in China should be thought of as a new phenomenon. Yet this is so. It is popularly believed, for example, that homosexually active young men learn this behaviour from foreign films, videos, books and magazines, from the 'sexual liberation' that is supposedly characteristic of the West. This has had important consequences for the way in which AIDS has been understood, for it too is widely seen as having been imported from outside. Although this is never written down as the official position on these matters, the authorities see gay men as a kind of social enemy, in that they are believed to be the main source of HIV infection in the country. This response is as much conditioned by political need as it is by any lack of understanding, just as it was in the past. Recently, medical workers carrying out HIV prevention education among behaviourally homosexual men have had their work halted (Wan, 1993).

### Homosexuality or Bisexuality?

The term 'homosexuality' is currently translated in Chinese as *tong xing lian*. This is a relatively new term in the Chinese language, appearing for the first time around 1911, just after the end of the last dynasty. Before then, there was no special term to describe sex between men. The description offered depended on what they were doing, the same words being used to describe both homosexual and heterosexual behaviour. In Chinese, four kinds of description are of relevance to homosexual behaviour between men, although the same phraseology is often used to describe heterosexual behaviour as well. First, there is a description for anal sex – *hou ting hua* – meaning literally 'to plant a flower in the back yard'. Second, there is *chui xiao* which describes oral sex when it is performed on a man by either another man or a woman. The literal meaning of *chui xiao* is 'to play a vertical bamboo flute'. Third, there are regional terms for masturbation be it performed by the man himself, or by a male or female partner. In north-eastern China, the term used is *lu gan*, meaning 'stroking a pole'. To describe anal sex between two men, the term *hao nan feng* is used.

Historically homosexuality and heterosexuality have never been considered polar opposites. Instead, homosexual and heterosexual behaviour were considered two parallel ways in which the same individual could gain sexual relief. This becomes evident through even a cursory reading of ancient Chinese literature in which every 'homosexual' character displays heterosexual behaviour, either at the same time or afterwards. For example, the two heroes in the literary work *Bian Er Chai*, which is perhaps the only pre-eighteenth-century homosexual novel, had had sex with women. Viewed behaviourally, the so-called male homosexuals of Chinese classical literature would seem to have been bisexual, as were many of the women in these same accounts.

In order to better appreciate how this could be, it may be helpful to consider the influence of yin-yang philosophy on popular beliefs about sexual behaviour in China. Just as everything is divided into yin and yang, so yin and yang can be changed into each other. Sexual behaviour between two men was popularly understood as involving the yang (male) man being transformed into yin (female) while having sex. Tolerant attitudes towards homosexual behaviour traditionally found in China derive from this. However, because of strong traditions of ancestry worship, non-procreative sexual behaviour was seen as a temporary substitute for heterosexual relations, a way of gaining sexual pleasure but not a means of ensuring generational continuity. Because of this, homosexual behaviour has never been accorded the status of hetero- sexual behaviour, even though it has been widely accepted.

Of course this does not mean that in China there have never been any men who are exclusively homosexual in their behaviour; there clearly are such. What it does suggest is that *society* tends only to recognize heterosexual and bisexual behaviour in men. Even today, the term used to describe sex between two men, and which is translated from the English – *tong xin lian* – still describes men's sexual *behaviour*, even though *lian* means love. In modern Chinese, *tong xin lian* is in fact an intransitive verb consisting of a present participle and a noun that is descriptive of the behaviour. If one wishes to ascribe identity to the person involved, the suffix *zhe* has to be added, as if to say 'homosexuality-er' in English. As for the idea that there might be bisexual individuals, this is much newer in Chinese. Traditionally, there has been no such description, and the translation for 'a bisexual man' – *shuang xin lian zhe* – is unfamiliar and largely incomprehensible to the majority of Chinese people.

These problems arise, at least in part, because until recently Chinese researchers and news reporters, even those who may be gay or bisexual themselves, have not had the opportunity to discuss bisexuality and homo- sexuality nor to draw distinctions between homosexual behaviour and homo- sexual identity.

### Contemporary Patterns of Behaviour

In recent years, a number of surveys have been conducted to examine patterns of sex behaviour among men who have sex with other men in China. Meth- odologically, however, many of these investigations are very weak, providing but partial insight into patterns of same-sex and opposite-sex behaviour. A recent survey of sexual behaviour among women and men attending sexual counselling sessions in connection with their reported homosexuality re- vealed that 63.5 per cent of the men were behaviourally bisexual (Lu, 1992). A questionnaire survey of 111 homosexual women and men (the sex ratio is not stated) revealed that 5 per cent were married, 21 per cent were divorced and 4 per cent lived apart from their spouse at the time of the survey (Gan, 1992). A recent survey of male homosexual activity in four large cities in China (reported on in detail later) collected data from 165 men, 46.7 per cent of whom reported they had sex with men only, 29.7 per cent reported they had sex with men mainly and with women occasionally, 9.1 per cent reported they had sex with men and women about equally, and 14.5 per cent reported they usually had sex with women but had sex with men occasionally (Pan, 1993).

A non-probability sample survey recently conducted in six provinces found that 0.5 per cent of married men living in cities reported lifetime homosexual experience, compared to 2.3 per cent of married men in rural areas (Liu, 1992). A recent random sample survey of university students in Beijing, however, found that among male students, 29.2 per cent reported having some homosexual feelings or experience, and 16.6 per cent reported having had a physical sexual experience with another male (Pan, 1994); 8.4 per cent felt themselves to be predominantly homosexual, and of these, 15.3 per cent reported having had sexual intercourse with a woman.

It has recently been estimated that in Beijing there may be between 10,000 and 20,000 men who actively participate in the homosexual social scene (Li, 1992). Several thousand of these men regularly visit the places where men go to find sexual partners such as the Dong Dan Park, Nan He Yan and San Li He. In Shanghai it has been estimated that there are tens of thousands of men who are predominantly behaviourally homosexual (Gan, 1992). This same study reported that the preferred location for having sex was the respondent's own home (60 per cent), specific hotels (29 per cent), in public parks (7 per cent) and public toilets (4 per cent).

In every big city there are places where behaviourally homosexual men meet. It is possible to identify at least fifty-four such locations in Beijing, forty-one of which are currently used, five extensively. In a recent field-based study, Pan and Wu (1993) visited twenty-three such locations in Beijing, Tianjin, Chongqing and Nanjing, including parks and toilets. In the course of the fieldwork, 810 men were contacted, of whom 188 declined to be interviewed. Of the remainder who were interviewed, 197 welcomed the opportunity to talk for fifteen minutes or more. Of the men in this study, 13.9 per cent lived in a city other than the one in which they were interviewed, or in an adjoining rural area.

### Preliminary Enquiry into Patterns of Male Bisexuality and Homosexuality in China

In the remainder of this chapter, we will report in more detail on findings from a preliminary enquiry recently conducted among behaviourally bisexual and homosexual men in Beijing, Tianjin, Chongqing and Nanjing (Pan and Wu, 1993, 1994a, 1994b). In-depth data were collected from 165 men as part of this work. They were recruited in parks, near public toilets and in other places where men meet to find prospective male sexual partners. Each was asked to complete a written questionnaire either on the spot (sixty men agreed to do this) or more privately and returned by mail. The mean age of respondents was 29.1 (s.d. 8.4). Seventeen per cent had received under nine years of education, 34.5 per cent had received between nine and twelve years, 22.4 per cent between thirteen and fourteen years, and 26.1 per cent more than fourteen years. Occupationally, 22.4 per cent were manual workers or labourers, 33.3 per cent were office workers, 21.2 per cent were professionals and 23.4 per cent were involved in other occupations.

For the purposes of the investigation, each man was nominally allocated to one of two groups depending on whether or not he reported having had penetrative sexual intercourse with a woman. Men who reported having done so were allocated to the lifetime bisexual group (53.3 per cent of the total sample), others were allocated to the exclusively homosexual group (46.7 per cent of the sample). Of men in the first group, 55.7 per cent reported mainly having sex with men and only occasionally with women; 17.0 per cent reported having sex with men and women approximately equally often; and 27.3 per cent reported having sex mainly with women and only occasionally with men.

### Reported Sexual Behaviour

Mutual masturbation and oral sex were the most frequently reported sexual behaviours in the last month among both groups of men, followed by anal sex (both receptive and insertive) and anilingus (see Table 11.1).

Relatively high numbers of male sexual partners were reported by both groups of men, as can be seen from the data in Table 11.2. Significant regional differences emerged in terms of the lifetime number of male partners reported, and the number of male partners in the previous month. Men in

*Table 11.1 Reported Sexual Behaviour*

| Behaviour | Lifetime | | | Last month | |
|---|---|---|---|---|---|
| | % Ever | % Never | No response | % | Mean reported frequency* |
| Kissing | 86.7 | 9.1 | 4.2 | 56.4 | 6.2 (N = 74) |
| Masturbating another | 93.9 | 1.8 | 4.2 | 56.4 | 6.0 (N = 79) |
| Being masturbated | 93.9 | 2.4 | 3.6 | 57.0 | 7.4 (N = 73) |
| Receptive oral sex | 75.2 | 20.0 | 4.8 | 42.2 | 3.3 (N = 59) |
| Insertive oral sex | 75.8 | 18.2 | 6.1 | 42.4 | 3.2 (N = 61) |
| Receiving anilingus | 50.3 | 43.6 | 6.1 | 18.8 | 3.3 (N = 27) |
| Giving anilingus | 24.2 | 69.7 | 6.1 | 7.3 | 3.2 (N = 11) |
| Receptive anal sex | 48.5 | 46.1 | 5.5 | 23.6 | 2.7 (N = 38) |

*The Ns reported in this column vary since not all respondents provided information on the frequency with which they had participated in each sexual act in the last month. Data in all other columns are for the whole sample (N = 165).

*Table 11.2 Mean Reported Number of Sexual Partners*

|  | Behaviourally bisexual men | Exclusively homosexual men | Significance |
|---|---|---|---|
| Lifetime | 39.3 | 96.8 | p = 0.0000 |
| Previous year | 10.2 | 24.4 | p = 0.0000 |

Tianjin and Chongqing, for example, reported having higher numbers of such partners than men in Beijing and Nanjing (p = 0.036 and p = 0.040 respectively).

Overall, 12.1 per cent of respondents reported not having a current sexual relationship with either a man or a woman, 33.3 per cent reported having an on-going sexual relationship with one person only, and 54.5 per cent reported currently having sexual relationships with more than one person. Of those in a relationship, 31 per cent met their regular sexual partner daily, 29 per cent at least once a week, and 40 per cent once a month or at longer intervals. Twenty per cent of respondents believed that their partner(s) only had sex with themselves, 33.3 per cent knew that their partners had sex with other people too, and 46.7 per cent did not know whether or not their partner(s) had sexual relation(s) with others. At the same time, 21.8 per cent were strongly opposed to their partners having sex with other people, 13.3 per cent were partly opposed, and 64.9 per cent had no clear feelings about the matter or had not considered the question before. Among those men who reported having a concomitant long-term sexual relationship, 77.9 per cent reported having had sex outside this relationship, and 72.1 per cent reported doing so in the last month. Of the men in the sample, 19.4 per cent reported having paid for sex at least once, and 18.2 per cent reported receiving money in return for having sex.

For lifetime bisexual men, those whose first sexual intercourse had been with a man reported having had their first sexual experience earlier (mean age 18.1) than those whose first sexual intercourse had been with a woman (mean age 19.3, p = 0.0000). Men whose behaviour was exclusively homosexual reported first having sex at an earlier age than those who had had sex with both women and men (p = 0.0282). Such a finding parallels that from a recent study of sexual behaviour among university students in China. Here, it was found that among male students reporting having had sex with other men, mean age at first intercourse was lower than that for their exclusively heterosexual counterparts – 17.1 years compared with 19.6 years respectively (Pan, 1994).

Among those behaviourally bisexual who were married, those whose first sex had been with another man reported higher numbers of premarital sexual partners than those whose first reported sexual experience had been with a woman. Of the former, 52.7 per cent reported having had more than ten premarital sexual partners, compared with 18.8 per cent of the latter (p = 0.0000). Behaviourally bisexual men whose first sexual experience had been with another man also reported knowing that sexual partner for a shorter period of time on average than those whose first sexual experience had been with a woman.

A relatively clear-cut relationship was found to exist, within this small sample at least, between the sex of the first sexual partner, and subsequent patterns of behaviour. Of all respondents whose first sexual experience had been with another man, 57.4 per cent reported being exclusively behaviourally homosexual thereafter, 71.3 per cent were involved in a sexual relationship with another man at the time of data collection, and 71.3 per cent reported having had no sex with a woman in the last year. Of men whose first sexual experience had been with a woman, the equivalent percentages were 5.3, 31.6 and 44.7 respectively (p = 0.0000, 0.0000 and 0.0060).

When the reported numbers of sexual partners of exclusively homosexual and behaviourally bisexual men were compared, it became clear that the men in the former group reported having significantly more lifetime sexual partners and partners in the last year than men in the latter – a mean of 105.5 compared with 68.8 (p = 0.0000) for lifetime sexual partners, and 24.6 compared with 10.6 (p = 0.0000) for sexual partners in the last year. Behaviourally bisexual men were also likely to report having had more male than female sexual partners – a lifetime mean of 39.3 male partners compared with 3.7 female partners (p = 0.000), and a mean of 3.0 male partners in the last month compared with 1.3 female partners (p = 0.0014).

Eighty-seven per cent of the exclusively homosexual men and 88.6 per cent of the behaviourally bisexual men surveyed reported having a regular sexual partner, even though they might also have other more occasional sexual relationships as well. Of those men whose regular partnership was with another man, 54.6 per cent reported having other partners as well. Only 8.2 per cent of men whose regular partner was a man felt it wrong to have multiple sexual partners, compared with 52.1 per cent of men whose regular partner was a woman (p = 0.000). Of men in a regular partnership with another man, 53.6 per cent reported that this relationship had lasted for one year or more, compared with 75 per cent of men in a regular partnership with a woman (p = 0.0000). The two groups did not, however, differ significantly in terms of the frequency with which they met their regular sexual partner, the frequency with which they reported having had sexual intercourse with this partner in the last month, and whether they knew if their partner had sex with others.

If we examine more closely the relationship between age at first sexual intercourse and the sex of the person concerned, an interesting finding emerges. Of those men reporting having had their first sexual experience between 16 and 20 years of age, 85.7 per cent report having had this first experience with another man. Of those who report first having sex after the age of 20, 47.7 per cent report having such sex with a woman. This may be a reflection of strong injunctions in Chinese society discouraging heterosexual intercourse outside marriage.

While we should be cautious in the interpretation of these findings, particularly given the relatively opportunistic way in which data was collected, there is some evidence that reported exclusive homosexual behaviour may vary by age. In this study, of respondents aged under 26, 66.7 per cent described themselves as exclusively homosexual, compared with 42 per cent of 26-to-30-year-olds, and 18.6 per cent of men aged over 30.


### HIV-Related and AIDS-Related Awareness

Respondents' overall awareness of AIDS was good. Only one respondent reported not having heard of AIDS, and responses to questions concerning the ways in which HIV is transmitted were reasonably accurate. Uncertainty and confusion was found to exist, however, in relation to blood transfusions and the possibility of acquiring infection through drinking from the same cup or from touching others (see Table 11.3). This suggests that, for this group of men anyway, there may be no clear-cut relationship between awareness of the routes through which HIV can be transmitted, and the means by which it is *not*.

Respondents were also reasonably knowledgeable about other STDs, and 15.8 per cent reported having had at least one such infection. As has often been reported in other studies, no direct relationship could be found between knowledge of STDs and HIV/AIDS and reported sexual practices. No statistically significant associations could be found between HIV-related knowledge

*Table 11.3 Perceived Routes of HIV Transmission*

| Mode of transmission | Correct response | Do not know | Incorrect response |
| --- | --- | --- | --- |
| Transfusing blood to others | 37.0 | 34.5 | 28.5 |
| Sharing the same cup | 47.3 | 27.3 | 25.5 |
| Touching an infected person | 64.2 | 24.2 | 11.5 |
| Through sexual intercourse | 80.6 | 18.8 | 0.6 |
| Through blood contact | 87.9 | 10.3 | 1.8 |
| Through sharing needles | 88.5 | 9.7 | 1.8 |

and current relationship status, reported numbers of sexual partners, and patterns of reported sexual behaviour. Rates of reported condom use were, however, higher than those for the population as a whole: 40.6 per cent of the men reported having used a condom in the last year and 19.4 per cent in the last month, compared with an overall mean of less than 10 per cent for the population as a whole (Pan and Wu, 1993).

Attitudes towards condoms correlated strongly with reported condom use. Among men who agreed with the statement 'using a condom is likely to make the penis go soft', 78.8 per cent had never used one, whereas among those who disagreed, 62.8 per cent had used condoms (p = 0.000). Condom availability seemed also to be related to condom use. Of those who were not sure where to obtain condoms, 76.4 per cent had never used them. Of those who reported obtaining condoms from relatives and friends, 77.8 per cent had used them at least once, compared with 61.4 per cent of those who obtained them in stores, markets and pharmacies, and 54 per cent of those who obtained them from hospitals or family planning centres (p = 0.000). Such variations may be related to the fact that in China, people (and young people in particular) may be anxious about obtaining condoms in public situations where they might be seen by others. Such anxiety persists in spite of government efforts to promote family planning in every hospital and work unit, and through every residential committee.

Regional variations were also found in reported rates of condom use, condom use being higher in Beijing (67 per cent) than in Nanjing (36.4 per cent), where reported usage was higher than in Tianjin and Chongqing, where it was around 25 per cent. Table 11.4 shows the percentage of respondents indicating agreement with a number of statements concerning condoms

*Table 11.4 Attitudes towards Condoms and Condom Use*

| Attitudes | Agree (%) | Ranked importance as a predictor of use |
|---|---|---|
| Using a condom makes you lose your erection | 31.5 | 1 |
| Condoms can slip off in your partner's body | 10.9 | 5 |
| Condoms reduce sexual pleasure | 50.3 | 6 |
| Condoms are easy to use | 60.0 | 9 |
| Men like their partners to put a condom on them | 32.7 | 10 |
| I will use a condom if my partner asks | 64.2 | 21 |
| Condoms can prevent STDs | 83.6 | 26 |
| No condom, no sex | 67.3 | – |
| Using condoms makes your partner unhappy | 10.3 | – |

and condom use, and the relative importance of each factor in predicting overall condom use using Akaike's Information criterion (AIC).

Overall, 37.6 per cent of respondents felt themselves to be at little or no risk of acquiring HIV, 37 per cent felt at some risk and 25.5 per cent had no idea. In bivariate analyses, personal perceptions of risk were found to be related to experience of anal sex. Of men who reported having had anal sex, 66.1 per cent felt themselves to be at some risk of becoming infected, compared with only 34.3 per cent of men who had never had anal sex (p = 0.0000). Frequency of reported anal sex in the last month was also an important predictor of personal perceptions of risk. For men who reported never having had anal sex, having had it once in the last month, and having had it more than once in the last month, the percentage who felt they were at no risk of acquiring HIV infection fell from 48.1 per cent to 23.8 per cent to zero (p = 0.0003).

Other factors predictive of heightened personal perceptions of risk included length of sexual relationship (p = 0.0003, the longer the relationship, the less the perceived risk), knowledge of whether or not a partner has sex with other people (p = 0.0016), having received payment for sex (p = 0.0003), and numbers of current sexual partners (p = 0.0058). The following factors were, however, unrelated to risk perception: demographic variables such as age, job and educational level, knowledge of AIDS, and the frequency of reading newspapers, listening to the radio and watching television.

### Sexual Behaviour Change

Only 30.3 per cent of respondents indicated that they felt it appropriate to modify their sexual behaviour so as to reduce the risk of acquiring HIV, 36.4 per cent felt that no change was necessary and 33.3 per cent did not know whether a change was necessary. In regression analysis, one of the most important predictors of positive attitudes towards behaviour change was agreement with the statement 'I would use a condom if my partner asked me to do so' (p = 0.001). Other factors predictive of such attitudes included being behaviourally bisexual – behaviourally bisexual men were more likely than exclusively homosexual men to express positive attitudes towards sexual risk reduction (p = 0.0025) – and holding strong religious or political beliefs (e.g. Confucian, Taoist, Buddhist or Marxist beliefs) (p = 0.0044). It is interesting to observe that the factors most strongly predictive of personal perceptions of risk are not identical with those best predictive of positive attitudes towards sexual behaviour change, suggesting that interventions to reduce risk among behaviourally bisexual and homosexual men in China may require complex and perhaps multi-staged interventions.

**Conclusions**

This chapter has discussed findings from a recent enquiry into sexual activity between men in China. It has highlighted the continued existence of such behaviour in circumstances where there may sometimes be official resistance to the acknowledgment of homosexual and bisexual behaviour among men. Traditionally, such forms of behaviour have long existed in China, although they have never been linked to what might be described as modern gay identities. Further enquiry will shed light on the meanings associated with male homosexual and bisexual behaviour, both for the actors involved and for Chinese society more generally. Access to such meanings will be essential for the design of effective interventions for HIV prevention that speak to the lived experience of the men concerned, addressing them in ways that seem appropriate and meaningful.

In the interim, there is evidence to suggest that while risk-related sexual behaviour between men takes place, knowledge about HIV and other STDs is generally good, relatively low-risk sexual practices such as masturbation and oral sex are among the most popular forms of sex, and attitudes towards condom use are not uniformly unfavourable. Indeed, there is some evidence from this preliminary study to suggest that condoms may be used when available, and in circumstances where the partner suggests them. Further enquiry is needed to further explore these and related issues, and the intervention options that flow from them.

**References**

BUTTERFIELD, F. (1982) *China: Alive in the Bitter Sea*, New York, Bantam Books/New York Times Books.

GAN, X. (1992) 'Homosexuals' Pathogeny and their Latent Harm to Health, Based on 111 Cases in Shanghai', *China Sexology*, 2, pp. 40–3.

GIL, V. (1991) 'An Ethnography of HIV/AIDS and Sexuality in the People's Republic of China', *Journal of Sex Research*, 28, 4, pp. 521–37.

GIL, V. (1992) 'The Cut Sleeve Revisited: A Brief Ethnographic Interview with a Male Homosexual in Mainland', *Journal of Sex Research*, 29, 4, pp. 569–77.

HINSCH, B. (1990) *Passions of the Cut Sleeve: The Male Homosexual Tradition in China*, Berkeley, University of California Press.

LAU, M. P. and NG, M. L. (1989) 'Homosexual in Chinese Culture', *Medicine and Psychiatry*, 12, pp. 465–88.

LI, Y. (1992) *Their World – Male Homosexual Group in Beijing*, Taiyuan, Shanxi Publishing House.

LIU, D. (1992) *Sexual Culture in Modern China*, Shanghai, Sanlian Publishing House.

Lu, L. (1992) 'Medical Analysis of 1,000 Homosexuals in Psychological Clinics', *China Psychological Health*, 2, pp. 112–15.

PAN, G. (1947) 'Causes of Homosexuality in Chinese Documents and Literature', in ELLIS, H. (Ed.) *Psychology of Sex* (1947 translation), Beijing, Sanlian Publishing House.

PAN, S. (1988) *Social History of Sexuality*, Zhengzhou, Henan People's Publishing House.

PAN, S. (1993) 'Sexuality in Current China', *Research in Sociology*, 2, pp. 76–85.

PAN, S. (1994) 'Random Sampling Survey on Students' Sexual Behaviour from Colleges and Universities in Beijing City', *Youth Research*, 5, pp. 124–32.

PAN, S. and WU, Z. (1993) 'Partnerships in Male Homosexually Social Activities', *Youth Research*, 12, pp. 45–9.

PAN, S. and WU, Z. (1994a) 'AIDS Risk in Male Homosexually Social Activities', *Zhejian Xuekan (Science in Zhejiang Province)*, 5, pp. 66–9.

PAN, S. and WU, Z. ( 1994b) 'Comparative Study between Male Bisexuality and Homosexuality', *Research in Sociology*, 6, pp. 58–62.

RUAN, F. F. (1991) *Sex in China: Studies in Sexology in Chinese Culture*, New York, Plenum Press.

RUAN, F. F. and TSAI, Y. (1988) 'Male Homosexuality in the Traditional Chinese Literature', *Journal of Homosexuality*, 14, pp. 21–3.

STAFFORD, P. (1967) *Sexual Behaviour in the Communist World*, New York, The Julian Press.

VAN GULICK, R. H. (1961) *Sexual Life in Ancient China*, Leiden, Holland, E. J. Brill.

WAN, Y. (1993) 'Some Thoughts on AIDS Education for Gay Men', unpublished manuscript, Beijing, National Health Education Institute.

ZHANG, B. (1994) *Homosexual Love*, Jinan, Shandong Science and Technical Publishing House.

Chapter 12

# The Homosexual Context of Heterosexual Practice in Papua New Guinea

*Carol L. Jenkins*

The purpose of this chapter is to discuss a form of sexual behaviour found among the peoples of Papua New Guinea which is not immediately understandable either to outsiders or to many Papua New Guineans themselves. The term bisexuality, as used elsewhere, may not cover all the variants in practice and conception discussed here. Some variants appear similar to forms found in other parts of the world and some do not. An analysis of the form of a sexual act, however, marginalizes the meaning of the act to its participants and to others in the society in question. In this discussion, while forms will be described, the major effort will be focused on attempting to understand what these behaviours mean to those who participate in them and to those who observe or otherwise come to know about them. Secondarily, the discussion will explore how HIV prevention could be enriched by a better understanding of the variation in sexual practices and attitudes found in Papua New Guinea.

Bisexual is the commonly used term to gloss aspects of the behaviour to be discussed here. Specifically, the current issue is male bisexuality. 'Bi', which means two, usually implies switching between opposite-sex object choices and same-sex object choices, actions notwithstanding. While the term has always been problematic, bisexual is still the term used in epidemiological and social studies of risk factors for sexually transmitted diseases (STDs) when the author wishes to refer to people who have sexual relations with persons of their own sex as well as with persons of the opposite sex. In particular, a concern has often been expressed that men who are bisexual may 'bridge' the heterosexual and male homosexual sub-populations. In so-called pattern one countries, where the AIDS epidemic appears to have begun and continues to predominate among behaviourally homosexual men, the possibility of a bisexual 'bridging' of transmission into the larger heterosexual sub-population is thought to be a real danger (Morse *et al.*, 1991; Tielman *et al.*, 1991). The fluidity with which some male sex workers move between paying and non-paying, male and female categories of partners, for example, as found on the island of Bali (Ford *et al.*, 1993) suggests that other types of 'bridging' transmission may be possible as well. In any event, the anomalous human being who seeks out and enjoys sex with persons of both sexes continues to baffle those who see themselves as falling neatly into one of two common categories, the hetero or the homo.

## Taxonomy and Relevance

The use of bipolar categories is universal in human societies, and the attempt to mediate the polarity by introducing a third term is not unusual. Yet conceiving of sexuality as a cultural domain which requires taxonomic efforts is rather new, and decidedly Western. The traditional peoples of Papua New Guinea generally did not have specific terms to designate one type of sexual orientation as opposed to another, although a term suggestive of an altered gender identity can be found in at least a few of the nation's 868 or more languages. In one location where pseudo-hermaphroditism is not uncommon, there is a specific term referring to the condition (Imperato-McGinley *et al.*, 1991), but the term may not reflect on gender or sexual orientation. In modern Melanesian Pidgin, a few descriptive terms reflective of homosexual orientation and/or preference are now in use, for example, '*geli-geli*' or '*tanim man*'. Others, such as '*poofter*', are largely derived from Australian usage and have pejorative overtones.

In general, sexual identity is not a contested issue in Papua New Guinea. The forces of culture which shape sexuality seem to have been configured in such a way as to leave a great deal of flexibility in desire and its agencies for human beings born with male genitals. For humans born with female genitals, the story has been quite different. There is simply no way to discuss bisexuality without taking account of the vast differences in the way in which sexuality is allowed to emerge, develop, and eventually mature in males as opposed to females in much of Papua New Guinea. Because socially prescribed gender traits may influence erotic preference and lifestyle choices, it is important to reiterate that females are far more often disadvantaged *vis-à-vis* males on any of a wide number of counts. Although there is ample evidence that females, young and old, do find avenues of self-expression not entirely under male control, in most Papua New Guinean cultures this requires a struggle against the taken-for-granted right of males to dominate and control females, especially in the areas of life surrounding sexuality.

Another important point to be made here is that specified and delineated sexual categories have little relevance to the real essences of sex as experienced and thought about by Papua New Guineans (and, I suspect, by a great many of the rest of us). These real essences are social, erotic, emotional, moral and ethical and, perhaps for some, magical. The actual sexual act is often of secondary significance and the gender of the participants may not play the critical role it does in many other sexual cultures; certainly, not a critical role in the attribution of sexual identities. This latter fact is sometimes difficult to see due to the widespread influence of European and American Christian belief systems which have altered remembered history. These have created embarrassment and shame concerning homosexual desires that were definitely not present in many pre-Christian New Guinea traditions.

### Transgression and Social Change

That which might be considered transgressive sex differs across cultures in Papua New Guinea and, as elsewhere, for some persons, may be the more delicious the more transgressive it is. In Papua New Guinea, as a general rule, transgression is more likely to adhere to the setting and the relationships among the participants in an act, than to the act itself. There are certainly rules about proper sexual conduct in every Papua New Guinean society, or there were. This latter remark is more than sarcastic. The rate and nature of historical change in Papua New Guinea is remarkable, although not evenly experienced across all cultural domains or geographical regions. There is no other major population group on earth which has experienced a shift from Neolithic technology and its associated sociocultural forms to an economy dependent on satellites and computers in so recent and short a time period.

What the effects have been on sexuality, the social contexts of sexual behaviour, complex ideologies of sex and gender, the institutions of marriage and family are not well known. Few societies were well described early enough to have a pre-missionary ethnographic baseline; even fewer of these have had a contemporary re-study to examine effects of modernization on sex and gender issues. The few that have include the Gahuku (Read, 1965, 1986), the Huli (Glasse, 1965; Clark, 1993) and a few others. It is clear, however, that where sexual customs (and mortuary customs as well) offended European observers, these could be suppressed into deep hiding very quickly (Parkinson, 1907). Our knowledge, therefore, of what the true range of sexual and reproductive beliefs and behaviours may have been at the time of contact is quite limited.

The ethnographic record demonstrates that some Papua New Guinean societies were strongly puritanical and repressive traditionally, while others were much more permissive. The myth of the golden age of sexual restraint circulates among Papua New Guinea's elders (as elsewhere) and almost every man and woman older than 40 in an opportunistic sample of over 400 persons interviewed throughout the nation in 1991 believed that sexual behaviour had increased in licentiousness. This conviction has nearly become a national dogma with major implications for the planning and design of HIV prevention programmes.

The evidence from ethnographic sources reveals a far more complex picture. It is clear, for example, that women were not aware of some male ritual homosexual practices existing earlier that had been kept hidden from them. It is also apparent that certain regimes of traditional permissiveness, where they were supported by religious ideologies of growth and fertility, have undergone the imposition of greater restrictions in modern times, as among the Kiwai, Gogodala and several Sepik peoples. In others, it is indeed likely that the breakdown of male initiation rites and the loss of associated social controls inhibiting heterosexual activity have led to greater, or at least more open, sexual activity among youth and adults alike, as among several of the peoples of the Eastern Highlands.

Nor is there any dearth of contemporary change agents to add to the powerful forces of church, state and the cash economy active in the past half-century. The newer change agents include a wide variety of fundamentalist, charismatic Christian sects, AIDS, AIDS researchers, pornography, satellite TV, comic books, literacy and formal education, Asian businessmen and others.

Hence, learning what the rules are about proper sexual conduct is not especially easy. This is most marked in urban settlements, some of which have in them persons from over 110 different language groups (Matasororo, 1994). Most of these persons would have moved into an urban centre from a mark-edly contrastive rural lifestyle within the past thirty-five years. An increasing proportion of the urban population is made up of young adults who have been born and raised in the city, who have rarely or never seen their '*asples*' (home village) and who do not know how to speak the language of either parent, speaking Melanesian Pidgin instead. Thus, a consensus on the rules or meanings in sexuality is not likely to be easy to find, on the topic of bisexuality or on any other.

## Methods and Materials

In order to make a first approximation at describing the behavioural domain of bisexuality as it might be configured in Papua New Guinea, I shall draw on the rich material collected by interviewers as part of a series of studies on sexual behaviour and risks of STD/HIV conducted between 1991 and 1995 by the Papua New Guinea Institute of Medical Research (Jenkins, 1994a, 1994b; The National Sex and Reproduction Research Team and Jenkins, 1994). None of these studies specifically sought information on bisexuality, but whatever personal experiences were reported as part of the interview were simply recorded. Some studies are on-going; at last count, more than 1,000 interviews on various aspects of sex and reproduction had been collected. Group sex (multiple men with one or few females) and same-sex activities were queried more directly than bisexuality in most studies. In addition, I personally conducted interviews with three specific men who, during their lives, have had more than casual sexual involvements with persons of both sexes, sometimes simultaneously. Where the relevant published literature exists, comparisons are made with collected descriptions and the interpreta-tions at hand.

### Dual Sexuality: Ritual and Male Cults

It is important first to clarify ritual homosexuality and its relationship to the topic of bisexuality. Numerous books and articles have been written on ritual homosexuality, both as case studies (Van Baal, 1966; Herdt, 1981) and in more comparative or theoretical frameworks (Herdt, 1984; Knauft, 1993). It is useful to distinguish secret male cults in which homosexual acts were obligatory and prescribed, as opposed to those in which the philosophical and emotional ambience encouraged heterosexual avoidance, sometimes to an intense degree, but did not set up homosexual liaisons as a matter of prescribed ritual.

In the culture area sometimes referred to as 'the semen belt' (southwestern region), the ideological underpinnings to ritualized homosexual practices usually centred on the sacredness of semen. The sacralization of body fluids is philosophically the flipside of the belief that a body fluid, even the same one, can be polluting, dangerous and even lethal. This is not simple bipolarity, but a dynamic sense that the goodness or badness of an object (act or attitude) is situational. For example, in the same culture in which a man's semen must be 'fed' to his sister's son so that the boy might grow into a man, that same semen, given to his wife during the last trimester of pregnancy or while the infant is breastfeeding, is thought to bring sickness or even death to the man's own offspring. A further point is that, in some of these societies, sexual rituals included plural heterosexual intercourse as well as homosexual rites. These were religiously justified acts to ensure the fertility of land and clan, to heal and to keep the ancestors happy. Only slightly different were the beliefs of the Angan peoples (and several of the Great Papuan Plateau groups as well), among whom it was thought that semen stimulated the growth of boys who, therefore, were inseminated orally, anally or by anointment, as the society saw fit. In these societies, homosexual and/or public, group heterosexual intercourse were required by custom.

The term bisexual, as used in contemporary epidemiology, does not seem well suited to what men experienced in these societies. In the course of their lives, all initiated men in these societies developed and maintained a dual sexuality. This allowed them to play the roles necessary to fulfil the ideals of manhood in their particular social systems, which sometimes required sexual intercourse with males, sometimes with females and sometimes with females in large male, public groups. Eroticism, for the individual, did not always adhere to each situation, making performance at times difficult (Van Baal, 1966; Herdt and Stoller, 1990). In recently collected sexual life history narratives, men from the regions in which these rituals once existed discussed them explicitly as customs of the past. One elderly man from the Papuan Coast stated clearly that he did not enjoy the anal sex rituals of his culture. Herdt (1981) also found that some men were frightened and even repulsed by the obligatory same-sex oral insemination rituals of their region. Others in these regions appeared to engage in all the required sexual activities with little protest and move relatively easily from one mode to the next. These are fairly gross impressions, however, given the scant ethnographic investigations carried out when the practices were still common.

In any case, these were unusual cultural forms by world standards, found in only a minority of New Guinean societies. Most of these societies were themselves quite small, rarely numbering over 6,000 persons. They were found within the Great Papuan Plateau and south-western coastal area from about Kikori to the Digul River in Irian Jaya, with another major node among the Angan peoples in the eastern end of the Highlands. Ritualized homosexuality was reported from other parts of Island Melanesia, but its distribution was limited when Europeans first reached the islands, even though, if theoretical reconstructions are correct, it may have been more widespread further back in prehistory (Herdt, 1984; Lindenbaum, 1984).

Homosexual rituals were in fact practised by a small proportion of Papua New Guineans, far fewer persons than implied by the claim that there is evidence of ritualized homosexuality in 10–20 per cent of all Melanesian cultures (Herdt, 1984, p. 56). More critically, these ritual complexes are nearly totally extinct today and are not important to discussions of HIV transmission or prevention or even to discussions of contemporary sexuality. They remain important, however, for several reasons. Firstly, in some areas where homosexual rituals once existed, non-ritual homosexual relations were also important (Ernst, 1991). If there were evidence to suggest that social attitudes toward homosexuality in those societies remain more permissive than elsewhere, there may be implications for HIV prevention. It has been observed that young male sex workers in Port Moresby are frequently from Papuan coastal societies which did have ritualized homosexuality or whose neighbours did (Jenkins, 1994a). More recently, however, young Highlands men have joined them, demonstrating that the promise of money is sufficient as a motivator and that earlier customs of ritualized homosexuality are certainly not necessary to the recruitment of male sex workers today.

Beside the purely intellectual challenge of explaining unusual cultural forms, understanding Melanesia's various homosexual ritual complexes is also important because those regimes may be seen as the expressive extreme, the tip of the iceberg, as it were, of a configuration composed of similar bipolar, sexually antagonistic and homoerotic elements which has far greater geographic spread and affects a much larger number of people than did homosexual rituals themselves.

### Bisexuality: The Usual Forms

Before discussing what I believe is the most common but subtle form of bisexuality in Papua New Guinea, it should be shown that the more usually recognized forms of bisexuality are present also. The following excerpt is a simple, straightforward statement of a 30-year-old single man who is often a client of both male and female commercial sex workers:

> Here in Moresby I always have sex with women and young boys who want money. My payment is from K5 to K30 per person – man, woman, boy or girl. I never have any problem with the police or the community in which I live. I don't show this kind of activity where everyone else can see. I always play under cover and always teach my partners to use condoms when they have sex with me. They always do what I want them to do. I never had an STD. I have been involved with buying sex for more than four or five years now. I might have spent more than K2000–K3000 on sex alone during those years.

Another pattern which has been fairly common, particularly in urban Papua New Guinea, is well known to older residents and has even been recorded in a novel of the AIDS era (Krauth, 1990). This is a type of sexual patron-client relationship. This particular type of relationship may be part of the colonial history of Papua New Guinea. It has shifted of late towards greater monetization, as have many types of sexual relationships. Its classic formulation is something like this: a white man, whose full sexual preference is for other men, seduces (or is seduced by) a Papua New Guinean man who has a heterosexual public identity. The white man is usually older and more wealthy. The local man receives and gives sexual pleasure as well as money, gifts and a nice place in which to sleep, bathe and eat much of the time. He often brings friends who share the advantageous surroundings, if not his sexual partner. This relationship may become quite enduring with the patron paying for educational costs or other constructive investments, as well as expenses such as bail if his lover gets in a fight and ends up in jail. Over the duration of this relationship, which could last many years, either man may have sex with others, and the local man, in particular, is likely also to have sex with women. At one point it is usual that the younger man's parents will decide he has been running free too long and needs to settle down. He may be called back to the village and introduced to the wife for whom he has been marked. At one point in the marriage negotiations, the patron-lover is introduced to the parents and the bride. In the fashion of kinship-based societies, he is incorporated as 'uncle' or a similar term from that time on. The younger lover marries, continues to drop by his patron/lover/uncle's for sex, money and other hand-outs as needed, and the first male child born to his new marriage is named after the patron-lover.

The last pattern I will document here is one which demonstrates a fluid mixing of heterosexual and homosexual erotics. The following quotation comes from a 38-year-old, working, single mother of two children, in a special relationship with her boss:

> He always said he wanted two men to fuck a girl at the same time so I let him do that only if he agreed to my condition about putting out

half the money for my car. He agreed and we went to a resort one weekend and we fucked and fucked until I was exhausted. Then he fucked his friend up the ass while I watched and his friend fucked him while I watched. This was my first time to see homosexual sex take place and it's not as bad as people describe it, I mean it was mutual between the both of them. Yes, we used condoms for whatever we did together but not when they were fucking each other's asses. Because they didn't come inside the ass, they dropped their semen on top of the back and later rubbed their cocks on the semen that was already outside on the skin. I don't do this very often with the boss, but now he wants me for that kind of sex only and other girls for ordinary fucks.

The term bisexuality is usually used to include behaviours such as those in the previous examples.

### Homoerotic Heterosexuality

There is another sense in which the term bisexuality may take on additional meaning. In both the distant and recent past, a common and widespread cultural pattern was one in which boys underwent initiations in secret male cults in which they were taught the dangers of female pollution. Most of these cults also taught boys how to behave sexually, including how to seduce women, avoid menstrual contamination, maintain erections, or other aspects of proper performance as a man and the maintenance of sexual health. In a significant proportion of these initiation systems, penile incisions of some sort were carried out. On a national scale, this type of society predominated and, with modern transformations, continues to predominate today.

In this type of system, boys are not specifically taught a positive role for same-sex practices; nor are they taught strongly negative attitudes about same-sex practices. The issue is simply ignored. What is given considerable scope, however, is a physical, sensual, and emotional camaraderie which is brought into existence, in part, by pitting the boys as a group against their elders in the set of ritual actions. The female is objectified as the seductive, dangerous other. She is necessary, valuable but essentially tainted and therefore intimate relations of long duration with females should be avoided. Even where initiations speak to marital relations *per se*, young men are never advised to become companions to their wives. It is considered a sign of weakness and threatening of future sickness and misfortune should a man spend time with a woman for anything more than the pursuit of reproduction. Marital relations are presented generally as complementary roles embedded in larger kinship networks, the most important relations of which are between men. Issues of heterosexual eroticism, sexual engagement and other aspects of intimacy must be avoided in as much as male domination and control of fertility are the aims of the cult and, on the level of dogma, there is no breaching of male dominance.

But sexual dogma and ideology, while they may inspire glorious music and art, are not tightly correlated with actual sexual behaviour, either in relation to the cult activities or beyond them in daily life (Leavitt, 1991). Today the secret male cults are considerably diminished in power and do not annually initiate more than a few thousand young men in any region of the country. They have, however, not lost influence entirely and in many areas the philosophical teachings as well as the penile surgery and other manipulations still continue. In fact, several new types of penile surgery have been incorporated into the modern myths of masculinity and their practitioners carry these out in non-traditional, non-ritual settings in both urban and rural areas. What is the most pervasive and persistent aspect of the secret male cult in Papua New Guinea, even where all remnants of the cult as an institution have vanished, is the objective of maintaining male dominance over females, possibly, as many authors have pointed out, because masculinity in these societies is seen as so vulnerable.

### Bonding

The descriptions of traditional initiations do not demonstrate a formal process of age grade naming and commitment of allegiance, such as those described for parts of East Africa (Moore, 1976). Nor are the initiates able to bond together to help each other at moments of real trial or crisis during the initiations. Each young man is required to stand on his own at the most critical times. Nonetheless, the ritual process of becoming a man is dramatically symbolized and physically experienced as one among many, i.e. as a self, a person among '*wantoks*'. The '*wantok*' idiom here refers to a group of other males of the same village or other area of affinity. '*Wantoks*' shift according to the structure of the current reference group. One's '*wantoks*' might be of one's own clan, own village, own language group or even own province, depending on which sodality is required by the situation.

The functions of intense male bonding have been discussed and the obvious made clear. Langness (1974) pointed to the undeniable need of bonding for fighting, as living under the threat of attack from enemies was the standard situation in nearly all areas of the country prior to the advent of the colonial state. The trade-off between developing strong bonds among men as opposed to strong marital bonds is an obvious area for possible conflict (and creative cultural resolutions). One ethnological perspective might interpret the function of male bonding as part of the process by which relative rank is established in the group, itself a mechanism to reduce the frequency of violent fighting amongst males (De Waal, 1982). That male bonding contributes strongly to the maintenance of control over females is a foregone conclusion, from all points of view. Whatever these functions may have been in more traditional lifestyles, today male bonding has important sexual as well as protective and economic functions. Despite the overall decrease in warfare and hunting/fishing, masculine roles remain defensive and acquisitive, enjoined to economic and protective functions of the clan or its urban equivalents.

Boys learn what they know about sex largely from other boys, often those only a little older than themselves. Sharing one's sexual experiences with one's *wantoks* is an important activity which may take place in a variety of modes. The most common form early in life is through discussions, as when older boys tell the younger ones about their experiences. They may even make and view drawings together. Practising with each other through anal inter-course is not uncommon in several areas of the nation, both traditionally and today at boarding high schools. Sharing a pornographic magazine or video is another increasingly common mode of bonding, with the occasional move into dyadic or group mutual masturbation. Boys go out searching for girls together and men continue to do the same as adults. These activities among boys are hardly unique to Papua New Guinea. They take place among girls too, but in more veiled forms.

What appears to be unique to the sexual cultures of Papua New Guinea is the degree to which the sharing of experience moves away from secondary to primary experience, i.e. actually having sexual intercourse with a female partner in the presence of and in cooperation with several to many other males, leaving the possibility open for homosexual intercourse to take place at the same time. I wish to be very careful in making this statement in order that the reader, whether a Papua New Guinean or not, is aware that there is very little written on this topic from any other part of the world. It may be, of course, that group sex in a variety of forms, including those under discussion here, does occur widely in the world but without the probing eye of sex researchers, and has not yet come out of hiding.

### Forms and Meanings of Group Sex

Researchers elsewhere have explored the role of male groups in arousal and search behaviours, but, for example, among Thai men, after drinking to-gether and encouraging each other, the trip to the brothel ends with each man going to a different woman (VanLandingham *et al.*, 1993). On the other hand, Mexican–Americans may hire a prostitute for a group of men, calling the practice 'becoming milk brothers' (Magaña, 1991). Material on the nature and variety of sex work in India reveals that men may go to a prostitute together – they say, in order to save money (Shreedhar, 1994).

In the USA, group sex is known in the context of a rock band and its 'groupies', and that of the 'pulling train' of street and fraternity gangs (Sanday, 1990). In heterosexual pornographic presentations in Western na-tions, sexual fantasy more often entails groups composed of several females and one male. In the recent random survey in the USA, when asked if group sex was appealing, 13 per cent of men aged 18 to 50 and only 1 per cent of females answered positively (Laumann *et al.*, 1994). It appears, however, that group sex in the USA survey was construed to mean the shifting of sex partners in a setting which allowed men to fulfil their wish to increase partner numbers, i.e. exchange female partners among males. This seems to be a different reading of the term group sex as used in Papua New Guinea, India and elsewhere.

The multiplicity of forms in which group sex (or, as Berndt labelled it in 1962, 'plural copulation') takes place in Papua New Guinea is distinctly biased towards multiple-male/single-female configurations. This has been revealed clearly by many men who discussed these activities with male interviewers in our studies. Most events appear to fit the form described in the following excerpt from a 29-year-old married man with one child:

> Group sex is one thing when all the young fellows who go around together have turns on one women. That is if only one of us is lucky enough to get a girl out from the disco/video or six-to-six. She wouldn't know that we are having turns on her until we have gone to a place where there's no house or no people around and then we start having sex one after the other. We have agreed already that we'll be having turns so nobody complains and nobody pays her too.

Women interviewers have found it very difficult to elicit a personal experience of group sex from women. The main reason for this marked discrepancy between male and female reports on group sex is that many types of group sex would be considered rape or forced sex by Papua New Guinean women. The terms used in Melanesian Pidgin to gloss this type of sex are '*lainap*' (line-up), '*singel fail*' (single file), and occasionally '*4-lain*' or '*dip lain*' (deep lain). Understood by women as attacks (on the self, one's clan or other group) and frequently justified by men with claims of fair retribution for having 'lost face' because the woman rejected him or simply that she was available and unprotected, these attacks are suffered by women and coated with shame. Shame derives from a fully socially supported pair of axioms that the male sex drive is barely controllable and that it is the woman's responsibility to reduce opportunities for sexual arousal. This is to be done through avoidance of visual and other contact with males or, at the least, through respectable and demure behaviour.

There is a corollary to the generally accepted belief in the force of the male sex drive; that excessive stimulation, 'going crazy', can take place in both men and women and that people are then not really responsible for what they do. The event is defined, much like drunkenness, as time-out behaviour. Pornography, alcohol and marijuana are said to contribute to excessive stimulation. In the past it would appear that, at least for the Highlands, fighting and its attendant psychophysiological correlates provided the context for excessive stimulation, leading to group sex and/or rape (Berndt, 1962). In recent focus group surveys the institution of the disco or six-to-six is unfailingly associated with the breakdown of past sexual mores, greater stimulation and the increase in *lainap* (line-up) or rape.

A 34-year-old single village man described events thus:

> When we drink or smoke marijuana, we get a strong feeling about sex and so when we see chances around, we don't let it go because we are not normal. We have another pressure on us to do what we can avoid when we are in our normal minds. When we hear about a disco somewhere, we young boys smoke marijuana and drink and we are there. That is where the line-up thing is practised. Some go for second or third rounds. We make sure her clothes are destroyed right away. The first ones go and play around with their penis and have their penis erected and come in for the next round. Sometimes girls feel really bad but one thing they don't do is take us to court. They feel ashamed of themselves thinking that many people will point fingers at them and say they have been fucked by so many men. That is one reason why we are not taken to court. In this kind of situation, the number of men involved will depend on how many people saw the incident. That could involve five men to fifteen men. Old men and small boys of 11 or 12 years take part. The female has no choice because all the lot have seen others having sex with her so she just gives in.

The proportion of men over 16 who report having participated in some form of group sex is high, over half of all interviewed, and there is no culture area in which it is unknown. The patterns described cover the range from highly coercive and violent to situations in which women are described as willing, sometimes accepting pay and even encouraging of group sex.

No matter which context for group sex, the women are either designated as '*pamuks*' (promiscuous women or prostitutes) when the men tell the story or seen as booty in a victorious fight with another group. Stripped and thrown over a man's shoulders, she becomes the meat he feeds his troops. The idioms of speech for these events focus on eating, meat, food and the camaraderie of men. The men queue, watch the performance of the guy in front and take their turns, usually several times in a night. Impatience, hyperstimulation, desire, all combine and homosexual (usually anal) intercourse can take place simultaneously with little comment. Examples very similar to the following were recorded by Berndt (1962) over thirty years ago.

From a 40-year-old married man comes the following description of what can happen. It begins with a denial:

> There was not one time when I fucked another man's anus or he fucked my ass. I remember taking part in group sex, just once. We

ten men and a woman from the Sepik. Because the first man fucking the woman was taking a while, we just could not wait so one of us ended up inserting his cock into the ass hole of the man fucking the woman. We all ended up in a line fucking the ass hole of the person before us. We had one woman so we changed places every now and then so that we all took turns in fucking the woman. This took place in the city botanical garden.

One important concept is that of '*sans*' or chance. Having a chance to join in on a group event is not something to miss; some, especially the elders, who rarely have a chance for sex, will now have theirs; more successful, dominant men will give a chance to the less successful, who will owe them a reciprocal chance later or, at least, allegiance. The opportunity is taken to teach one's younger male relative (brother, cousin) about sex, even to holding his hips to teach him how to move. Instead of fighting over a woman, the men show their capacity to cooperate, enjoy each other's sexuality and totally ignore the woman.

Should there be any question of responsibility for the event (defined as rape or adultery), blame falls on a group, not on an individual. Complicity within the entire community in almost every event described was complete, including among other women who simply state that the victim is a '*pamuk*' or it is not their concern because she is not one of their relatives. Reports repeatedly state that males of all ages, from early puberty to aged, participate. In only a very few urban cases did the woman complain to legal authorities, usually naming the leader of the group or the one holding a major weapon.

A 29-year-old married man, with two children, living in an urban settlement, stated the following:

Many times I got a female, I take them into the vacant church and fuck them. After me, other boys who have seen the incident or who were around have chances (line-up). When they hear of us with a female, they creep out of their beds and spy. It is not young fellows only. All the males in the settlement are involved. From the youngest to the oldest in the block are involved. Whoever sees or hears about it and comes to the venue, they want to join in. They can't let the chances go. One time we were in this process when a young boy of around 12 or 13 went to have his chance when his turn came. I went there and touched his buttocks while he was in action. Later after ejaculation, he came and said to me, I urinated in the vagina. Actually he ejaculated but it was his first experience so he thought he urinated.

There are numerous examples of older men helping a younger man learn to have intercourse by physically participating in his experience, i.e. by holding on to his body or on to both the female and the male body. Commercial sex workers have explained that men frequently wish to buy sex for themselves and their buddies, a situation which usually costs more in Papua New Guinea. The homoerotic and, at times, frankly homosexual aspects of this type of heterosexual group sex is striking for its easy disregard of categories thought by some people to be more exclusive than they are. While far less frequently recounted, an opposite version also does take place in which one man and several women engage in group sex, with the women having sex with each other as well as with the man.

## Meanings and Implications for HIV/AIDS Prevention

The implications for HIV prevention are multiple and serious. In a recent study of sexual behaviour, among men who recounted exact numbers of persons involved, there were forty-four acts of group sex involving 52 women and 445 men (The National Sex and Reproduction Research Team and Jenkins, 1994). The tendency for Papua New Guinea men to enjoy sharing their sexual experiences with each other, even to the point of mixed homosexual-heterosexual events, raises the possibilities of exposure to in-fected body fluids, in this case, the semen of other men, by an average factor of at least eight. Even if no homosexual intercourse were to take place, this would remain true.

In that a very high proportion of group sex events appear to be coercive, against the woman's will, one might think that more rigorous enforcement of the law against rape would be of value to AIDS prevention in Papua New Guinea. Women, however, do not yet see the role they play in maintaining the reign of terror in which they live. It is unlikely much can be done to diminish the high frequency of rape until a significant number of women and at least a minority of men understand how and why this social form has such destruc-tive power.

Condom usage, however, is generally acceptable, even by rapists. Eye-witness accounts describe a proportion (never all) of participants in group sex, including those involved in alleged rape, using condoms. Bisexualities, of any of the types described, entail little risk of HIV infection if condoms are consistently used. Making condoms widely and easily available would appear to be the most direct and most effective public health intervention possible. Knowing the range of sexual styles engaged in also suggests that a variety of condoms could be sold, possibly including stronger ones for anal sex.

If a man acquired an HIV infection during a line-up, it is far more likely to be due to man-to-man transmission than to woman-to-man transmission. The homoerotic elements of the group interaction are masked by an apparent heterosexual context. Because of this masking, it is likely to be missed as a special risk for HIV acquisition and little prevention effort is likely to be targeted for group sex *per se*. The notion of bisexuality is too vague and linguistically ambiguous to describe any particular mode of transmission in Papua New Guinea, and possibly in other nations as well.

### References

BERNDT, R. (1962) *Excess and Restraint: Social Control among a New Guinea Mountain People*, Chicago, University of Chicago Press.

CLARK, J. (1993) 'Gold, Sex and Pollution: Male Illness and Myth at Mt. Kare, Papua New Guinea', *American Ethnologist*, 20, 4, pp. 747–57.

DE WAAL, F. B. M. (1982) *Chimpanzee Politics: Power and Sex among Apes*, New York, Harper & Row.

ERNST, T. (1991) 'Onabasulu Male Homosexuality: Cosmology, Affect and Prescribed Male Homosexual Activity among the Onabasulu of the Great Papuan Plateau', *Oceania*, 62, 1, pp. 1–11.

FORD, K., WIRWAN, D. N. and FAJANS, P. (1993) 'AIDS Knowledge, Condom Beliefs and Sexual Behaviour among Male Sex Workers and Male Tourist Clients in Bali, Indonesia', *Health Transition Review*, 3, 2, pp. 191–204.

GLASSE, R. (1965) 'The Huli of the Southern Highlands', in LAWRENCE, P. and MEGGITT, M. (Eds) *Gods, Ghosts and Men in Melanesia*, Melbourne, Oxford University Press.

HERDT, G. H. (1981) *Guardians of the Flutes*, New York, McGraw-Hill.

HERDT, G. H. (Ed.) (1984) *Ritualized Homosexuality in Melanesia*, Berkeley, University of California Press.

HERDT, G. H. and STOLLER, R. J. (1990) *Intimate Communications*, New York, Columbia University Press.

IMPERATO-MCGINLEY, J., MILLER, M., WILSON, J. D., PETERSON, R. E., SHACKLETON, C. and GAJDUSEK, D. C. (1991) 'A Cluster of Male Pseudohermaphrodites with 5α-Reductase Deficiency in Papua New Guinea', *Clinical Endocrinology*, 34, pp. 293–8.

JENKINS, C. (1994a) 'Behavioral Risk Assessment for HIV/AIDS Among Workers in the Transport Industry, PNG', report presented to AIDSCAP/FHI, Bangkok.

JENKINS, C. (1994b) 'Situational Assessment of Commercial Sex Workers in Urban PNG', report presented to Prevention Research Unit, Global Programme on AIDS, World Health Organization, Geneva.

KNAUFT, B. (1993) *South Coast New Guinea Cultures*, Cambridge, Cambridge University Press.

KRAUTH, N. (1990) *JF Was Here*, Sydney, Allen & Unwin.

LANGNESS, L. H. (1974) 'Ritual Power and Male Domination in the New Guinea Highlands', *Ethos*, 2, pp. 189–212.

LAUMANN, E. O., GAGNON, J. H., MICHAEL, R. T. and MICHAELS, S. (1994) *The Social Organization of Sexuality: Sexual Practices in the United States*, Chicago, University of Chicago Press.

LEAVITT, S. (1991) 'Sexual Ideology and Experience in a Papua New Guinea Society', *Social Science and Medicine*, 33, 8, pp. 897–907.

LINDENBAUM, S. (1984) 'Variations on a Sociosexual Theme in Melanesia', in HERDT, G. (Ed.) *Ritualized Homosexuality in Melanesia*, Berkeley, University of California Press.

MAGAÑA, J. R. (1991) 'Sex, Drugs and HIV: An Ethnographic Approach', *Social Science and Medicine*, 33, 1, pp. 5–9.

MATASORORO, E. (1994) 'New Government for NCD', *The Times*, Thursday 22 December, 781, 1, 3.

MOORE, S. F. (1976) 'The Secret of the Men: A Fiction of Chagga Initiation and its Relation to the Logic of Chagga Symbolism', *Africa*, 46, 4, pp. 357–70.

MORSE, E. V., SIMON, P. M., OSOFSKY, H. J., BALSON, P. M. and GAUMER, H. R. (1991) 'The Male Street Prostitute: A Vector for Transmission of HIV Infection into the Heterosexual World', *Social Science and Medicine*, 32, pp. 535–9.

THE NATIONAL SEX AND REPRODUCTION RESEARCH TEAM and JENKINS, C. (1994) *Papua New Guinea Institute of Medical Research Monograph No. 10*, Goroka, PNG Institute of Medical Research.

PARKINSON, R. (1907) *Dreissig Jahre in der Sudsee: Land und Leute, Sitten und Gebrauche im Bismarck Archipel und auf den duetschen Salmoninseln* (trans. N. C. BARRY, n.d.), Stuttgart, Strecker und Schröder.

READ, K. (1965) *The High Valley*, New York, Columbia University Press.

READ, K. (1986) *Return to the High Valley*, Berkeley, University of California Press.

SANDAY, P. R. (1990) *Fraternity Gang Rape*, New York, New York University Press.

SHREEDHAR, J. (1994) 'Behind Closed Doors', *World AIDS*, 36, 2.

TIELMAN, R., CARBALLO, M. and HENDRIKS, A. (Eds) (1991) *Bisexuality and HIV/AIDS: A Global Perspective*, New York, Prometheus.

VAN BAAL, J. (1966) *Dema, Description and Analysis of Marind-Anim Culture*, The Hague, Martinus Nijhoff.

VANLANDINGHAM, M. J., SUPRASERT, S., SITTITRAI, W., VADDHANAPHUTI, C. and GRANDJEAN, N. (1993) 'Sexual Activity among Never-Married Men in Northern Thailand', *Demography*, 30, 3, pp. 297–313.

## Chapter 13

## *Silahis*: Looking for the Missing Filipino Bisexual Male

*Michael L. Tan*

About two years ago, while processing questionnaire data gathered from 'men who have sex with men' attending HIV prevention workshops, I noticed that about a quarter of the participants self-identified as 'bisexual'. I found this strange since I had attended many of the workshops as a facilitator but rarely did I hear the participants speak about bisexuality and bisexual experiences.

I mentioned the data over dinner with a housemate, who had been a participant in one of the workshops, and asked, 'Where are all these *silahis*?', using a local slang word that loosely translates into 'bisexual'. My housemate smiled sheepishly, 'I'm one of them.' I was startled since I had always known this housemate to be 'homosexual', not 'bisexual', at least in terms of his dates and sexual partners. As things turned out, my friend had had girlfriends in the past and this included sexual relationships. He in fact could remember the exact date on which he first had sex with a woman, but could not give the date for his first sexual experience with a man. While he had not had sex with women for two years, he considered himself bisexual.

Having lived in the Philippines most of my life, I probably should have been prepared to understand the invisibility of bisexuals and, in general, the often tentative gender boundaries that contribute to this invisibility. My housemate's sheepish smile reminded me, too, about the awkwardness and unease that accompanies discussions of bisexuality, whether in relation to oneself or to others.

My interest in pursuing research on bisexuality in the Philippines grows out of my involvement with HIV/AIDS prevention projects. The epidemiology of the AIDS epidemic led Western researchers to coin a behaviourist term – men who have sex with men – that was supposedly neutral, to include people who did not necessarily self-identify as gay, homosexual, or bisexual. This approach has both its advantages and disadvantages. On one hand, it has allowed HIV prevention groups, at least in the Philippines, to reach people who would otherwise have been intimidated by labels of 'gay' or 'homosexual' in relation to educational materials or workshops. On the other hand, this approach reinforces the boundaries that prevent access to many shadow populations that do not see themselves as men 'having sex' with men. We will see that this is particularly the case for men involved in bisexual behaviour, men who in a sense defy existing norms not just of 'heterosexuality' but also of 'homosexuality' and are, in the process, further marginalized.

This chapter is mainly based on work with HIV prevention programmes with two non-governmental organizations: with the Library Foundation, a Manila-based gay men's organization that works with men who have sex with men, and with the Health Action Information Network's (HAIN) various HIV/STD prevention programmes, particularly with male sex workers. Much of this work has involved workshops using interpersonal health education approaches, i.e. intensive discussions of the psychosocial issues relating to HIV/AIDS. These discussions have often yielded rich information on sexual cultures in the Philippines.

I must emphasize that I have not been involved in a formal research project dealing with bisexuality and so the information is often derivative in nature, drawing from different projects as well as observations of popular culture. Teaching undergraduate and graduate courses in Sex and Culture at the University of the Philippines has provided additional opportunities to probe into sexual cultures. In retrospect, a project specifically dealing with bisexuality, or bisexualities, would probably have been nonsensical, given its diffused and elusive qualities.

In preparing this chapter it became clear that there is, in fact, no published work on bisexuality in the Philippines, although occasional passing references are made in papers on homosexuality. Understanding bisexuality will require more than what we have at present, which is still limited to Metro Manila. At the same time, one should not discount the role that mass media have played in developing a national sexual culture, certainly not integrated or totally consistent, but with many areas of consensus. I will first present an overview of the social and historical context of sexual culture in the Philippines. I will then review some of the surveys on sexual behaviour as they might relate to bisexuality. This will take us into the central discussion of the paper, focusing on the concept of *silahis* and their representation. The last part of the chapter will deal with public policy considerations in HIV prevention, as they relate to bisexual behaviour.

### Social and Historical Context

The Philippines lies on the eastern fringe of Asia, an archipelago of more than 7,000 islands. It went through more than 300 years (1571 to 1898) of Spanish colonization and nearly half a century (1898 to 1946) of US occupation. The colonial past has often been described in the media as '300 years in a convent and 50 years in Hollywood', a comparison that is sometimes used, obliquely, to explain sexual cultures in the country. This unfortunately glosses over the complex social forces that impact on sexual cultures.

Spain, for example, left more than Roman Catholicism and its authoritarian patriarchy. Spain also entrenched feudalism and its strong class distinctions. This stratification continues to influence many aspects of social life, including religion itself and, ultimately, sexual cultures. As for the influence of Hollywood, this certainly has not been in the form of hedonism; if anything, it comes in notions of romantic, maudlin love. Spanish religious culture actually found continuity in the erotophobic, fire-and-brimstone moralism of US Protestant evangelicals. At the same time, the US colonial occupation saw the introduction of more secular ideologies that were often as strident as their religious counterparts.

Among these secular ideologies were those of psychology and biomedicine. The Americans introduced the terms, and Western-based concepts, of 'heterosexuality', 'homosexuality' and 'bisexuality'. Filipinos are exposed to these concepts usually through schools and the media, and graft these on to older popular gender constructs, some of which have pre-colonial origins. The result can be highly syncretized concepts, as we see with the following gender constructs.

As in other Southeast Asian societies, male transgender categories continue to dominate the public's concept of a homosexual. In Tagalog (the basis for Filipino, the national language), the term used is *bakla*. The *bakla* – often a cross-dresser working as a beautician or dress designer – is foremost an effeminate male, which easily accommodates the popularized versions of Freudian Oedipus complex explanations of homosexuality: the dominant mother and the absent father. The *bakla* is distinguished from 'real men' (*tunay na lalake*); conversely, the *bakla* is, properly, sexually attracted to these 'real men' and not to other *bakla*.

The rise of gay consciousness in the West, particularly in the United States, has spilled over into countries such as the Philippines. The terms 'homosexual' and 'gay' are now used in many Philippine languages, usually as synonyms for *bakla*. Since the late 1980s, there has been some local gay activism, spurred in part by the HIV epidemic and the need to launch community-based prevention programmes. Still very much middle- and high-income based, some of the emerging gay communities self-identify as 'gay' as well as *bakla*, the latter term having been reappropriated much as 'queer' has in the United States and the United Kingdom. On the other hand, many middle-class Filipino men may identify as 'gay' but not as *bakla* because the latter are seen as low-income, effeminate males.

The term 'bisexual' is not as widely used as 'homosexual' but, as will be explained later, it does figure in public discourse. *Silahis* is a Tagalog term that is sometimes used, as slang, to refer loosely to bisexuals. Note that the term is almost exclusively used for males. While people acknowledge that a woman can be bisexual, they find it difficult to conceptualize a woman engaging in bisexual 'acts'. This reflects the traditional weaknesses in conceptualizing female sexuality, at least from the viewpoint of sexual acts. Curiously, indigenous linguistic equivalents for 'heterosexual' do not exist in any of the Philippine languages (or, for that matter, any of the Southeast Asian and East

Asian languages). Neither has the term 'heterosexual' been borrowed into local languages as 'homosexual' or 'bisexual' have. The term is rarely used colloquially and I have actually had several encounters with people who understand it to be 'another' perversion like 'homosexual' or 'bisexual'.

### Existing Quantitative Data

As in many other countries, quantitative research methodologies – mainly KABP (knowledge, attitudes, behaviour and practices) studies – dominate the field of HIV-related research in the Philippines. I have mixed feelings about such research. On one hand, numbers are needed for lobbying work with politicians and policy-makers. On the other hand, such numbers are all too often decontextualized, contributing to the reinforcement or even creation of public myths that sometimes become counter-productive. Reviewing some of these survey findings for insights on bisexuality will show the limits of this approach.

One survey, conducted in 1988–9, was commissioned by the US funded AIDSCOM project as part of its assistance for the Department of Health's AIDS programme. The survey was conducted by Trends, a marketing research firm, focusing on so-called sentinel populations that were viewed as possibly being at risk for HIV. The surveys were in the traditional KAP (knowledge, attitudes and practices) mode, using face-to-face interviews. Although not involved in the research design, I was asked, after the surveys were completed, to synthesize and analyse the findings.

Among 200 'men who have sex with men', recruited through convenience sampling and consisting mainly of self-identified homosexuals, 49 per cent reported that almost all their sex partners were 'straight males'. About a third of this group also reported having had sex with women. The Trends survey had many methodological problems. For example, the researchers still used archaic terms such as 'covert' and 'overt' homosexuals. The gender of sex partners, while interesting, does not shed light on perceptions about sexual identity.

In 1990, the World Health Organization (WHO) commissioned several surveys on partner relations in different countries. In the Philippines, the

*Table 13.1 Usual Gender of Sexual Partners of Males, Metro Manila*

| | |
|---|---|
| Female only | 92.2% |
| Mostly female, some male | 3.7% |
| Equally male/female | 0.3% |
| Mostly male, some female | – |
| Only with males | 3.1% |

*Source:* Tiglao, 1991.

study was conducted in Metro Manila, involving 1,670 randomly selected respondents aged 15 to 59. One section of the questionnaire was on the usual gender of the respondents' sexual partners. The findings for males are presented in Table 13.1.

Asking about the 'usual gender' of sexual partners has some utility, but remains limited in terms of what it can tell us about sexual identity. This is complicated by biases that may emerge from the use of particular data collection methodologies. In this survey, face-to-face interviewing was used, which could affect the reported number of same-sex partners.

In 1991 and 1993, the Health Action Information Network (HAIN) conducted surveys among health science students in Metro Manila, as part of baseline data gathering for HIV prevention workshops. These surveys asked students what their sexual orientation was. In this survey, we included definitions of 'heterosexual', 'homosexual' and 'bisexual' in terms of 'attraction' to 'the opposite sex', 'the same sex' and 'both sexes'.

The process used to draw definitions is itself useful for obtaining insights into the construction of sexualities in the Philippines. We added these definitions after a pre-test showed that there were students – even among those taking nursing – who did not understand what 'heterosexual' was. As I mentioned earlier, there is no Filipino word for 'heterosexual', but we presumed that the term was widely understood. When the pre-test showed this was not the case, we decided to retain the use of the English 'heterosexual' and to add on definitions in Filipino. This was where we realized how difficult it was to translate these constructs. If we had used actual sexual experience or behaviour, then we would have been left with many blank answers since many of the students had not had sexual intercourse. On the other hand, what was 'attraction'? And for 'bisexual', would we have to qualify 'equally attracted' or not as the Tiglao survey for WHO had done? Table 13.2 shows the summarized results from the two surveys.

Again, the numbers offer nothing certain. In fact, when we broke down the figures using different variables, more questions emerged. For example,

Table 13.2 *Self-Identified Sexual Orientation, Health Science Male Students*

|  | 1991 (N = 354) | 1993 (N = 133) |
|---|---|---|
| Heterosexual | 91.2% | 92.5% |
| Homosexual | 2.0% | 1.5% |
| Bisexual | 4.8% | 3.0% |
| Not sure/uncertain | 2.0% | 2.3% |

*Note*: The 1991 survey covered medical and nursing students. The 1993 survey covered students in dentistry, medical technology and midwifery.

*Table 13.3 Self-Identified Sexual Orientation and Sex Partners of Participants in HIV Prevention Workshops for Men Who Have Sex with Men (1993–4), The Library Foundation* (Reporting period: six months before the workshop)

| Homosexual (N = 143) | Sex partners | Bisexual (N = 53) |
|---|---|---|
| 116 | Males only | 36 |
| 6 | Male and female | 14 |
| 1 | Female only | 0 |
| 20 | No sex/no answer | 3 |

*Source*: Tan (1994).

we found that using income levels as a variable, the numbers of 'not sure/uncertain' rose as income levels dropped. The surveys with health science students also emphasized the need to understand that surveys with the 'general population' – including segments such as students, or young adults – will overlap with other groups such as men who have sex with men.

Accessing populations of men who have sex with men may be a bit more useful for reaching 'bisexuals'. The HIV prevention programme of The Library Foundation, a gay men's organization reaching men who have sex with men, offered such an opportunity. In the Foundation's HIV prevention workshops for men who have sex with men, about 25 per cent self-identify as 'bisexual' and 70 per cent as 'homosexual' in English questionnaires that they fill out at the start of the workshop. It is striking that the figures have remained almost fairly constant across twenty-two groups who have taken the workshops since the programme started in 1992. Nearly all of the participants in these workshops have college education and are fairly comfortable with English. The questionnaire only asked how the participant felt about what his sexual orientation was, without specifying what 'sexual orientation' might mean.

It is interesting how the labels for sexual orientation do not necessarily translate into sexual behaviour, at least in terms of sexual partners, as illustrated in Table 13.3. Note that among those who self-identify as homosexual, about 5 per cent had had sex with both men and women in the six months before the workshop, and one 'homosexual' participant had had sex only with a woman. Among those who self-identified as bisexual, about 68 per cent had had sex with men only, while 26 per cent had had sex with both men and women.

This brief review of available quantitative research shows both its potentials and limitations for the study of sexuality. The numbers are tantalizing, especially when different surveys yield similar figures. Yet the surveys have many limitations. For example, Sittitrai *et al.* (1991), commenting on findings from the WHO-sponsored Survey of Partner Relations in Thailand, point out the problems in analysing the data because of differences in definitions of such key terms as 'having sex'. The more formidable problem, however, is explaining what seem to be 'discrepancies', such as the information from The Library Foundation's men who have sex with men, where identities such as 'homosexual' and 'bisexual' do not necessarily correspond to actual sexual behaviour, at least in terms of choice of sexual partners. This is where qualitative research is important, not so much to provide validation of the quantitative research, as to question the conceptual frameworks of sexuality research in general.

### The Bisexual in Public Discourse

The quantitative data gave some insights into bisexual behaviour (in terms of sexual partners) and posed a few problems about bisexual identity and its relationship to bisexual behaviour. Understanding the construction of identity and behaviour requires an analysis of how bisexuality is described – or not described – in public discourse. In order to explore this in greater depth, I will focus on the word *silahis*, a Tagalog word that means 'rays of the sun' and which has, since the 1970s, been used as a loose gloss for the English 'bisexual'. It is now in use even in non-Tagalog areas, apparently integrated into national Filipino slang. The reasons for the choice of this word seem to have disappeared from discourse, although one older gay informant tells me – while qualifying that he is not sure either – that *silahis* is a metaphor referring to the change of identity a person has from 'day to night'. The etymology is not as important as the usage of the word. Here, I will focus on popular usage, including the contestations of meanings within and among different groups. I will describe usage among three 'groups': the 'general public', male sex workers, and the *bakla*, and analyse some of the more salient meanings of this discourse, including subtexts and semantic nuances.

### Perspectives from the 'General Public'

The term *silahis* is used fairly widely, mainly to refer to males who are 'attracted' both to males and females, a definition clearly derived from Western biomedical and psychology texts. Not surprisingly, in focus group discussions and classroom discussions with university students, other elicited synonyms are all in English: 'bisexual', 'ac/dc', 'double blade'. I have never been able to get a consensus on whether 'attraction' alone is sufficient, or whether one has to have sex with both men and women, in order to be 'bisexual'.

The popular perception of the *silahis* is that he is not *bakla*. He may have sex with other men, but he is not effeminate, at least not publicly so. One informant, Robert, who self-identifies as *bakla* and works in a large office, related to me how his officemates began to speculate about what he was. He was not dating women, and there were 'too many' phone calls coming in from men. The 'problem' was that Robert was not effeminate. The conclusion was that he 'probably' was *silahis*. Robert, who works in advertising, proposes a play on words: '*Silahis*. When you can't be sure.'

Class seems to play an important role in shaping perceptions. The popular perception is that the *bakla* is not just effeminate, but is also of the lower classes. A yuppie male can cross-dress and be called androgynous or hip, and if there are suspicions about his sexual partners being also male, then maybe he is *silahis*. There is actually little certainty in the public discourse about the *silahis*, mainly because he blends into the population at large. The interrogation of one's identity, that could lead to a *silahis* label, emerges mainly in the context of personal relations: officemates or students wondering about each other; girlfriends about their boyfriends and wives about their husbands; parents about their sons and, as we will see, men about themselves. *Silahis*, when it is applied, is rarely final. It is tentative, and therefore tense. It is, as Robert puts it, when you cannot be sure since, after all, one is never sure about sexual acts and partners.

## Perspectives from Male Sex Workers

The discourse surrounding sexual acts is important as we look into the male sex workers' use of the term *silahis*. In our HIV workshops, we ask male sex workers to categorize their clients. The categories are quite consistent: *bakla*, *silahis*, and *matrona*. *Matrona* refers to middle-aged women. The *bakla* is an effeminate person. The *silahis* actually forms the broadest category, functioning almost as an 'etcetera' or 'miscellaneous' label under which all other male clients would be classified. The *silahis* is the married client whose wife is away; the action star (actor) who 'becomes a woman in bed'; or the high-ranking government official who may or may not be married. The *silahis* is also described through linguistic hybrids: the *macho gay*, the *baklang hindi ladlad* (the closet *bakla*).

The discourse often revolves around clients. Once, I was asked by a group of male sex workers if a certain university professor was *bakla*. I asked why they were wondering and they explained: 'he was huge, like a military personnel'. I answered back, 'But this professor is married, and has kids.' The sex workers concluded: 'He's *silahis* then. Imagine, we thought he was *bakla* because his wrists kept flicking. But see, you are right – he's married and has kids. And that big body. He couldn't be *bakla*.'

In one small group discussion with male sex workers, I posed a hypothetical situation: how a *bakla* can tell if his lover is not another *bakla*, referring to the traditional taboos on *baklas* having sex with another *bakla*.

The discussions initially centred on sex acts. A true male (*tunay na lalake*), the sex workers proposed, would not take the passive role in anal sex, nor would he give a blow job. A true male, too, would take a long time to climax when having sex with another male. I took the hypothetical situation a step further by asking: 'What if someone did all that was expected of a "true male" but was the one who first proposed sex?' I posed the question knowing that a 'true male' is not allowed to make such a proposition for sex with another male. There was some discussion about this, discussion that suggested confusion. After all, this hypothetical person did everything right, except to propose sex. Finally, a consensus emerged: this person is not *bakla*, he probably is *silahis*.

The discussion was important in making another distinction, not just between the *silahis* and the *bakla* but also between the *silahis* and the *lalake*, the 'real man'. Among male sex workers, these gender constructs have greater 'verifiability' among that of the 'general population' since their reference to sexual acts is often based on actual engagement. Thus, a customer who is married 'must' be *silahis*. At the same time, verifiability is limited, constrained by other facets of existing gender ideologies such as who can or cannot propose sex. In such instances, the use of *silahis* falls back on Robert's proposition, a post facto label, when you can't be sure.

*Silahis*, for the male sex workers, represents a configuration of attributes, ranging from movements of the wrist to body size to marital status. There is some overlap in these concepts with those of the 'general population', but because the male sex workers have actual sexual experiences with the *silahis*, the attributes are expanded to include what one does or does not do in bed, and to get to bed. We will see later that the acts are actually inconsequential and that it is the social framing of these acts that, ultimately, informs the gender labelling process.

### Perspectives from the *Bakla*

We move now to the *bakla*, a more 'stable' category in terms of public perceptions as well as in self-perceptions. The *bakla* is visible – some will say, too visible – defying gender categories yet conforming to a stereotype of the feminized male. Among the *bakla*, the main point of contention is whether the *silahis* is really attracted to females. The tone is accusatory, almost scoffing as is often expressed as: '*Sila'y baklang hindi ladlad*' ('They are *bakla* who are not out').

There is, clearly, an element of resentment that comes with accusation. The *silahis* is not just 'not out' but does not want to come out. The *silahis*' masculinity, or his having a wife or girlfriend, is a front: *Nagpapalalake* (trying to be male). The *bakla*, who defiantly flaunts social norms, holds the *silahis* in contempt. The reasons for the contempt are complex and varied. Some of the reasons are rooted in what one might loosely call gay or *bakla* pride. Other reasons may border on misogyny as expressed in jokes about having sexual relations with women.

Assumption of the *silahis* role, or even a preference for a *silahis* sexual partner, must also be recognized and analysed in relation to other social tensions or contradictions. I have mentioned class discrimination being present in the construction of the *bakla*. The *bakla*, as I have mentioned earlier, is constructed as being low-income; thus, an upper-income man who has sex with men may distance himself from the *bakla* by calling himself *silahis*. In workshop discussions among yuppie gay men, there is a distinct preference for the *silahis*, which simultaneously expresses 'liberation' from stereotypes – not being limited to 'straight men' – but also declares one's non-interest in, or even aversion for, the lower-class *bakla*.

The example above, as it relates to 'attraction', shows how problematic the standard biomedical and psychological definitions are for homosexuality and bisexuality because *silahis* and *bakla* are not just self-ascribed terms but are also terms ascribed by others. I am 'not *bakla*' (and therefore am possibly *silahis*) because I am 'respectable', because I can be attractive to some junior executive who sees himself as gay. The point of attraction can be taken a step further, into an even more complicated domain of desire. Note that it is the same *bakla* who will, on occasion, declare that there is no such thing as a *silahis* but who will, on many other occasions, assert with great confidence that 'all Filipino males are bisexual'. The English 'bisexual' is used, invariably, and not *silahis*. If asked to explain, the *bakla* will switch linguistic codes and go '*Lahat na Pinoy, pa-make*' ('every Filipino male can be bedded [by a *bakla*]').

The *bakla*'s usage of *silahis* is clearly different from his usage of 'bisexual', the former being a category of a closet *bakla* and the latter referring to the potential, in terms of availability for sex, in every Filipino male. Yet the two terms find conceptual convergence in attraction and desire, even as they play on concepts of *lalake*, the male, and *pagkalalake*, masculinity. Rather than being self-ascribed identities, we find one's identity ascribed by other people's definitions. The *bakla*'s usage of 'bisexual' is one of 'when you want to be sure', only slightly different from the public's usage of *silahis*, couched in 'when you're not sure'.

### *Silahis* and Gender Ideology

So far, we have discussed popular definitions of *silahis* and have seen how these play on ambiguity and dubiousness, more often as perceived by others rather than by self. We have not looked into how the *silahis* defines himself. This presents methodological difficulties for research as we return to a basic epistemological question: is a *silahis* someone who identifies as such, or is the *silahis* to be behaviourally defined, regardless of self-definition?

A simple way out is to say that there is bisexual behaviour – men who have sex with both men and women – and that there are bisexuals, people with that identity, whatever ways it is constructed and defined. This approach does not, unfortunately, resolve the question of the *silahis*. One cannot speak, for example, of *silahis* behaviour as in the English 'bisexual behaviour'. If this were possible, then we could rely on the survey data cited earlier. The problems become even more complex if we attempt to use *silahis* as a gender construct, mainly because *silahis* itself reifies the transgression of gender boundaries.

One reason the *silahis* is elusive is because there is the lack of disclosure. We see in the various forms of public discourse that the concept of *silahis* revolves around gender behaviour, around what is 'essentially' male and female and the derivations of masculinity and femininity. The *bakla* is a pre-colonial stable category, foremost the feminine male. The sexual persona comes later, building around Western concepts of 'homosexuality'. The *silahis* defies the norms for 'heterosexual' males (grafted on to older concepts of 'real men') as well as those of the *bakla*. He has sex with other men but he is not effeminate. At least in public, he neither confirms nor denies his sexuality.

An alternative way of looking at the *silahis* is to think of *silahis* as a gender role embedded in a system of developing sexualities that in a sense become stages in life. In practical terms, the *silahis* may self-identify as such because he is socialized into that role. The following two cases clearly show this socialization process.

Lito was 17 when he first started having sexual relationships with other men. At about the same time, he began to date women. He is not sure if he ever found women attractive but dating women was 'the normal thing to do'. Later, he began having sexual relationships with women, again because this was 'the thing to do'. When he was 21, he got his girlfriend pregnant. He still supports the child, who is now 7 years old. He has not dated women in the last three years, and presently has a steady boyfriend. He considered himself *silahis*, but now identifies as *bakla*.

Bobby is 28 and has had an Australian male lover for five years now. Before meeting this Australian, he was 'occasionally' active with men but 'more frequently' with women. He is still sexually active with women, but says he is 'monogamous' with his male lover, who does not live in the Philippines and with whom he meets a few weeks in a year. He enjoys going out with gay men and to gay-oriented bars. He has *bakla* (which he defines as 'effeminate gay') friends but thinks it unlikely that he will have sex with them. He considers himself *silahis*, a term which he comfortably exchanges in conversations with the term bisexual.

The cases of Lito and Bobby, similar to that of the housemate I mentioned at the start of this chapter, show how *silahis* can represent an assumed role, based on who one sees or dates even without recognizing the social reasons – in many instances obligatory – for those dates. It should be pointed out that both Lito and Bobby are seen as 'masculine' or 'butch' by the gay community, which factors into the self-ascription of *silahis*. Precisely because it is a role, *silahis* may also not be assumed, as in the following two cases.

Mario is 25. His first sexual experience was with a male. Most of his sexual experiences have been with males and he now has a steady boyfriend. Prior to this boyfriend, he had a relationship lasting almost a year with a woman. The relationship was quite serious, including plans for a marriage and children.

Mario self-identifies as *bakla* and as gay. He is emphatic about not being *silahis*, even while he had his sexual relationship with a woman.

Edgar is in his early forties and is a well-known hairdresser. Edgar has two children: 'I did it to please my parents. I told them, "There, I've given you two grandchildren. That's it." ' He self-identifies as *bakla*.

Much has been said about men who have sex with men but self-identify as heterosexual or 'straight' (or, in the Filipino context, *lalake* or male). The cases of Mario and Edgar show how one can have sex with women and not identify as 'straight' or bisexual. Mario and Edgar are not necessarily subverting existing gender ideologies. Their identification as *bakla* is a choice of a stable gender category. *Silahis* is too ambiguous, almost ludicrous, especially when, as Mario describes it, 'one feels *bakla*'. Both Mario and Edgar are effeminate by local definitions and are, by virtue of that effeminacy, also ascribed as *bakla*. Sexual acts, and sexual partners, do not make for gender identity. One 'feels' he is *bakla*, or *silahis*. At the same time, we must recognize that 'feeling' is not completely subjective. Society still constructs what a *bakla* is, and tries to construct what a *silahis* is.

Early in 1995, The Library Foundation sponsored a small group discussion on sexual identity, giving ten hypothetical male characters of different ages, marital status and occupational backgrounds, accompanied by brief descriptions of their sexual lives. Participants in the discussion were asked to give their opinions about each of these characters, to be narrowed down to two: 'I'm sure' (to mean he is *bakla*) and '*Hindi*' (No, he is not *bakla*). *Bakla* was used loosely here to mean 'homosexual' or 'gay'. Participants were not allowed to say '*silahis*' or 'bisexual'.

The discussions showed how much consensus there could be, based on the most superficial of criteria. For example, '35, single, works in advertising' drew unanimous consensus: 'I'm sure.' More interesting were the areas where there was dissent, especially in the attempts to resolve the ambiguities. Thus, there was uncertainty about '18, college student, with girlfriend, sometimes goes to Jurassic (code name for a park with cruising) and does not ask for pay' the reason being he was still young. In contrast, '45, separated from his wife, with four kids, once picked up someone at Bat Cave (a cruising place), wants to repeat this' is 'definitely *bakla*', the reason being age – the younger the person is, the more room for unresolved sexualities. A young man having sex with another man could be doing it for fun, for curiosity. An older man 'knows' what he wants.

The exercise merely confirms a strong developmental aspect underlying the construction and ascription of sexuality in the Philippines. Age marks off points in life cycles that, in The Library Foundation's discussion, becomes vital in terms of 'knowing'. Thus, '10-year-old, teased constantly as *bakla* in an all-boys' school, does not know anything about sex' is not 'yet' *bakla*. 'Knowing' about sex is an added dimension. The element of attraction and desire takes root here and can be used to look at the cases presented earlier.

The Library Foundation's discussion group involved a group of men who self-identify as 'gay', dissecting what *bakla* is. The exercise did not refer to bisexuals, but does offer insights into perceptions of bisexuality in terms of the verdicts passed, for example, on married men who have sex with men.

Public perceptions probably are not that much different. There are young men, who self-identify as heterosexual, having sex with *bakla* and explain it as simply 'having fun' (*pa-happy-happy*). The *bakla* is an easy outlet, even providing some financial gain. Eventually, it is expected that these men will stop having sex with *bakla*. They are not considered by others, or by themselves, as *bakla* or *silahis*. These instances of situational bisexuality are well-documented in the literature.

In other cases, relations with the *bakla* may be maintained in what has been called Latin bisexuality (Parker, 1989). As long as a 'male role' is maintained both sexually (as in being the insertor in anal intercourse) as well as non-sexually (not doing the laundry, or not cooking), such males are considered males or *lalake*, not *bakla*, not *silahis*.

On the other hand, we have seen the case of Lito, who goes through a period of 'obligatory bisexuality' or, in Ross' (1991) taxonomy, 'defense bisexuality' in his youth because he is socialized into that role. Self-identifying as *silahis*, in his youth, represents an accommodation. How he is perceived is another matter: by other *bakla*, he may be considered as a closet queen, while his girlfriends considered him 'a normal man' (Lito's terms).

The problem with existing taxonomies of bisexuality or bisexualities is that they remain compartmentalized, almost as if the labels represent discrete categories. In reality, there are instances where the different categories may merge. For example, the categories of situational bisexuality and Latin bisexuality often overlap, not just in sexually segregated communities such as prisons but also in settings where there may in fact be choices. An example comes with construction sites, where male workers share living quarters. Access to women is present, but there may be a choice to take on what has been described in Brazil as 'solidarity sex', an aspect of male camaraderie. In such situations, the men remain *lalake*. Eufracio Abaya (1994), a Filipino anthropologist currently doing work on the *bakla* in 'rurban' (rural-urban) areas, has found beer-drinking – traditionally an arena for socialization among 'real men' – to be expropriated by *bakla* for socializing with these 'real men' and leading to sexual encounters.

The norms of maleness, of machismo and of being *lalake*, are important. We have seen how this is operationalized in 'solidarity sex', where men can have sex with men and remain 'male'. It is in this context that we look again at the *silahis*. The *silahis* represents a transition. He is not *bakla* but neither is he *lalake*. Western definitions of bisexuality centre on sexual partner choice. *Silahis* may not even consider that choice. In many cases, we will have men who have had sex only with men and who would be classified as 'homosexual' in a Western framework and yet be *silahis* in the Philippines simply because they do not fit into the stereotype of an effeminate male. I described earlier the case of Robert, a yuppie gay man who is not, in fact, effeminate, but self-

*219*

identifies as *bakla*, a result of an emerging politicized gay community. Robert's officemates, cosmopolitan yuppies as they may be, are unable to understand how one can like men and not be like a *bakla*. Here, *silahis* comes after the fact, a label that resolves cognitive dissonance even as it leaves unanswered questions of 'sexual orientation' and 'sexual identity'.

### Sexual Ideology and *Silahis*

The relationship between gender ideologies and the construction of the *silahis* role is often quite apparent. Less obvious are the ways in which gender roles interact in diverse social arenas and the ways in which the interactions are shaped by broader sexual ideologies.

I have described two cases, those of Mario and Edgar, involving two *baklas* who have had sexual relationships with women but retain their self-identification as *bakla*. Their cases illustrate the importance of understanding how sexual ideologies shape *silahis* as a role. In the Philippines, one has to understand how the reproductive imperative – and its relationship to marriage and family – becomes an overarching theme in a dominant sexual ideology. Particularly in rural and semi-urban areas, children are produced not just as a duty but as part of 'becoming fully a person' (Abaya, personal communication). Marriage and children are investments for old-age companionship and care. Reproduction has nothing to do with sexual orientation. This explains why the *bakla* as well as gay men often 'fade' away from the social scene, usually after the age of 30, to raise a family. They do not necessarily stop sexual activity with other men; in fact, quite often this becomes clandestine activity, sometimes with sex workers.

Marriage can transform the *bakla*'s status in his local community, especially when he becomes *tatay*, a father. Becoming a father is the 'natural' thing to do; otherwise, one is *sayang*, wasted. The hairdresser, Edgar, who is quite visible in the media, stirs hopes among parents of *baklas*: 'If he can do it, so can you.' The potential for breeding is paramount. One yuppie *bakla* relates how his mother has tried to convince him to marry after watching Edgar on television: 'For all you know, you'll like it. Edgar's so much more effeminate than you are. Who knows, maybe you're a latent bisexual.'

Marriage is important because it offers some hope of 'conversion'. While Filipino fathers believe they can beat the man out of a *bakla*, mothers think marriage is the solution. Reyes (1989) has reviewed the depiction of homosexuality in Filipino films and notes that one of the recurring themes is that of women being seen as 'a cure for homosexuality', whether by dragging a young *bakla* to the whorehouse or by getting older *bakla* to marry. Most significantly, many of the scripts for these films are produced by *bakla* themselves. This is not done tongue-in-cheek – interviews and focus group discussions among *bakla* consistently show marriage as a viable goal, 'some time after 30'.

Marriage and child-bearing can bring major shifts in ascriptions. In Abaya's research in a semi-urban area, the *bakla* who marries is now *de pamilya* (of a family). There are new generic role expectations: he has to be more responsible now, providing for the family. But there are also expectations that he will not be as *pabakla-bakla*, as effeminate, as swishy. His new status is neither *bakla*, nor *silahis*, even if he continues to have sex with men.

At the same time, in other areas, mainly urban, marriage and child-bearing can be redeeming, but not necessarily redemptive. The *bakla* will often still be called *bakla* and, in many cases, the child of a *bakla* becomes the object of taunting from other children. Being effeminate is unacceptable and if the *bakla* father is known to continue to have sex with other men, social ostracism and contempt become even more strident. In fact, the discrimination against the *bakla* father is an expression both of machismo and of misogyny – pressured into becoming a father, the *bakla* is now expected to be male, as a father would. To remain *bakla* – by effeminate behaviour, or by having sex with other men – is contemptuous because it is to assume the role of a woman, which is incongruous with his being a father.

What is intriguing is that the social construction of, and attitudes towards, the *silahis* father are different. The *silahis* is not effeminate. Therefore the transition to the reproductive imperative may not be as radical. Opinions are mixed about the *silahis* father. Seen as being at least masculine, the *silahis'* sexual acts may not be deemed as transgressive, or deviant, as those of the *bakla*. On the other hand, precisely because the *silahis* is constructed as being masculine, his having sex with other men – while married to a woman – can be perceived as more deceptive and heinous.

We see here the importance of understanding the social contexts in which gender identities and roles develop. In Western terms, the married *bakla* and *silahis* are both bisexuals. Sexual cultures in the Philippines show otherwise: the two are different even if both move into 'bisexuality' (as sexual acts) under the same impetus: the reproductive imperative that comes with the dominant sexual ideology.

### I'm Sure!

*Silahis* is ambiguous. Yet when a *bakla* is asked if he thinks so-and-so is *silahis*, he will go, 'I'm sure.' 'I'm sure,' accompanied by raised eyebrows (*taas kilay*), has many meanings ranging from mild doubts to complete incredulity. In many ways, 'I'm sure' captures so much of the public's construction of the bisexual. The *bakla* does not believe the *silahis* exists; the average man or woman on the street believes he exists, by virtue of gender dogma. He is *silahis* because he cannot be *bakla*, either because he has children, or because he is not effeminate, or both. Affirming that someone is *silahis* then becomes a leap of faith.

The *silahis* therefore shuttles between two worlds, with connotations of potential deception and betrayal. The *bakla* whose partner is a *silahis* frets that he will eventually go for a woman. 'Straight' men – carrying stereotypes of the homosexual as predator – wonder about their best friends, their drinking partners. Women fret about their boyfriends and husbands possibly being bisexual, or gay (the distinction probably does not matter). Margarita Gosingco Holmes, a clinical psychologist who once had a popular newspaper sex advice column, says that she received many letters from women who have 'doubts' about their boyfriends. One letter, published in Holmes' (1994) collection of columns dealing with homosexuality, is worth reproducing in full:

> I have a boyfriend who is in his early 30's. We kiss, we hug each other, but we don't have sex. I, for one, prefer to wait until after marriage to have sex. But I am bothered with the way my boyfriend acts. Sometimes, when he walks, when he places his hands on his hips, when his lower lip drops, when he waves his hand, when he reacts after we kiss – are action/acts which are common to homosexuals. How would we know that a man is a homosexual? A bisexual? Or a man merely effeminate in his ways.
>
> If a man is one of these, can there be a problem in our sexual lives later? When we kiss, he has a hard on; does this mean he can still perform a sexual act even if he is one of the above?

The letter is signed 'Scorpio '91', and captures so much of the public construction and perception of the *silahis*. Scorpio '91 starts out by saying she has never had sex with her boyfriend, which comes through almost as an accusation even if she is quick to qualify that she prefers it that way. Scorpio '91 seems to be aware that a man can be 'merely effeminate in his ways' but frets, nevertheless, because any 'one of the above' may be a transgression, may create a problem in their future sexual life.

It is interesting that this shuttling between worlds in fact problematizes *silahis* as identity. *Silahis* becomes relational: he is one thing to his *bakla* partner, and another to his girlfriend or wife, and still another to a fellow *silahis*. Scorpio's letter also shows that the *silahis*' association with the *bakla* (and with other *silahis*) makes him a shadow of a shadow population. The *silahis* does not draw jesting and taunting like a *bakla* does. Because the *silahis* is a shadow role, it is one difficult to attack or even to confront. The coming-out process for a *bakla* is described as *pagladlad*, literally translated as an unfurling of one's cape. It is dramatic and flamboyant. A *silahis*, on the other hand, never makes *ladlad*. In the rare cases of disclosure, it is a process of *nabuking*, of being found out, of being exposed, thus the almost obsessive search – by girlfriends and boyfriends – for clues, for 'signs'. Disclosure here is never voluntary, *buking* being a verb always used in the passive tense. More significantly, one is not found out as a *silahis*. In many Filipino films, the wife who discovers her husband is seeing another man will confront him and scream, in spiteful rage, '*Bakla*'. Disbelief is resolved through accusation, not of the *silahis* but of the *bakla*. In a way, we come full circle in our discussion: the *bakla* thinks the *silahis* is a closet *bakla*, finding convergence with the enraged wife's final accusation, upon forced disclosure.

### Implications for HIV/AIDS Programmes

About 20 per cent of cumulative reported HIV cases in the Philippines are attributed to 'homosexual/bisexual transmission'. Unlike Western countries, the Philippines has not seen much gay scapegoating and homophobia directly associated with the AIDS epidemic, although violence against the *bakla* has always existed, contrary to Western descriptions of 'tolerance' of homosexuality.

Until recently, all of the Filipinos with HIV who had gone public were women sex workers. In 1994, two Filipino men came out, both saying they were bisexual. It is not clear how these two Filipinos will impact public discourse on bisexuality. Neither project themselves as *bakla*. One said he had sex more often with women than with men and he believed he had been infected through a woman sex worker. The other says he is married and has two children, and claims he was infected through a 'gay lover'.

Parker *et al.* (1991) have written about the need to describe sexual culture in terms of distinctions 'between cultural ideals vs. actual practice, public vs. private conduct, and prescribed vs. voluntary behaviour'. The representations of *silahis* show how important it is to describe such distinctions. We have seen how *silahis* may in fact be a social role, ascribed – by self or by others – at various stages in the life cycle with varying meanings. It is ambiguous because it is derived both from the rigidity of gender role expectations, particularly those relating to masculinity, as well as the potential for subverting that rigidity. We have seen, too, how *silahis* might or might not be assumed in different social contexts and life stages, and how this relates to sexual ideologies. Its use revolves around social desirability, allowing a shuttling across sexualities and sexual acts. Unlike 'bisexual' in the Western biomedical framework, with its fixation on sexual partner choice, the sense of gender identity in *silahis* is much more complicated, drawing from while transforming sexual and gender ideologies.

Unlike the *bakla* and the emerging gay communities, the *silahis* is often isolated, a shadow of other shadow populations. This has both advantages and disadvantages. On one hand, the *silahis* is not as easily taunted and persecuted as the more visible *bakla*. On the other hand, the *silahis* is isolated, often without even a peer group of other *silahis* to whom to relate. Social support, including HIV prevention programmes, will be harder to establish given that discrimination against bisexuals often comes not just from 'heterosexuals' but also from the *bakla* and gay men.

Establishing specific HIV prevention programmes for 'bisexuals' will be unrealistic, given the diversity of bisexualities that exist. At the same time, the *silahis* is pervasive, an expression of dominant sexual ideologies of masculinity, marriage, and reproduction. Great caution is therefore needed when working out information and educational materials for undifferentiated audiences of men who have sex with men. The use of materials with homoerotic themes, for example, may not be appropriate for people who adopt the *silahis* role and its underlying sexual ideologies.

I started this chapter by referring to The Library Foundation's HIV prevention workshops for men who have sex with men. It is significant that a quarter of the participants in these workshops self-identify as bisexuals. These workshops began mainly among people who self-identified as 'gay', suggesting that the sexual networks can extend from one sexual culture to another. Note that while participants in these workshops can use pseudonyms when they register, attendance at the workshops does involve some risks in terms of disclosure. One could continue with the exercises in semantics and speculate if a *silahis* remains a *silahis* after participating in these workshops, given that the social construction of *silahis* is so anchored on non-disclosure.

There are signs that changes are taking place. Elsewhere (Tan, 1994), I have discussed how emerging 'gay' identities draw from the traditional *bakla* construct. Similarly, there seems to be an evolution from *silahis*, as a role, to a kind of 'bisexual-ism' that draws on both indigenous, traditional culture and a global, cosmopolitan sexual culture. It is expressed, for example, among yuppie men who have sex with men as a preference for 'other bisexuals' rather than the *bakla*. Underlying this preference is still a traditional preference for the 'masculine' even as it flaunts the taboos on sex among 'gay' men. Being bisexual in this context has no reference at all to reproduction or marriage; instead, the preference for men and for women seem to revolve around sexual attraction, built on traditional social arenas. This emerging 'bisexuality' remains limited, mainly to middle- and high-income men in Metro Manila. It is interesting how, among these men, the term 'bisexual' is used, rather than *silahis*, almost as if *silahis* is left to its traditional meanings, together with its ambiguity.

The AIDS epidemic has catalysed gay community organizing efforts in several urban areas in the Philippines. Such organizing, with extensive networking and occasional mass media exposure, will eventually impact on sexual cultures. This will lead to a reframing of perspectives and concepts. For example, the term 'men who have sex with men' occasionally appears in the popular media and I have heard quite a number of 'gay' men asking each other, 'Do you think so-and-so is an MSM?' Such developments will, undoubtedly, affect Filipino 'bisexuals', whether they see themselves as *bakla*, *silahis*, bisexual, or 'straight'.

Earlier, we saw the case of Mario, who has sex with both men and women but self-identifies as *bakla*, assumed here almost as a political identity, of belonging to an organized community that is gay in a Western sense. But Mario himself admits that if a 'bisexual' or *silahis* support group existed, he probably would have assumed such an identity. Mario's case hints at what could happen, given specific conditions both locally and internationally. The notion, for example, of a 'support group' derives both from Western trends of self-help groups and from local norms of small group affiliation.

The future of 'bisexuals' and 'bisexuality' in the Philippines – as with 'homosexual' and 'homosexuality' – will depend on many social and cultural factors that impact on the formation of sexual cultures. Some of these shifts, such as growing urbanization, are predictable while others, such as the tensions between religious fundamentalism and secularization, are more difficult to project. Taken a step further, the impact of these changes need to be seen in relation to changes in gender and sexual ideologies. This will include changes in the emerging global sexual cultures and the expanding linkages among groups organizing around alternative sexualities.

## References

ABAYA, E. (1994) personal communication.

CARRIER, J. M. (1980) 'Homosexual Behaviour in Cross-Cultural Perspective', in MARMOR, J. (Ed.) *Homosexual Behaviour*, New York, Basic Books.

HOLMES, M. G. (1994) *A Different Love*, Pasig, Anvil Publishing.

PARKER, R. (1989) 'Bodies and Pleasures: On the Construction of Erotic Meanings in Brozil', *Anthropology and Humanism Quarterly*, 14, pp. 58–64.

PARKER, R. G., HERDT, G. and CARBALLO, M. (1991) 'Sexual Culture, HIV Transmission, and AIDS Research', *Journal of Sex Research*, 28, 1, pp. 77–98.

REYES, E. A. (1989) *Notes on Philippine Cinema*, Manila, De La Salle University Press.

ROSS, M. (1991) 'A Taxonomy of Global Behaviour', in TIELMAN, R., CARBALLO, M. and HENDRIKS, A. (Eds) *Bisexuality and HIV/AIDS: A Global Perspective*, New York, Prometheus.

SITTITRAI, W., BROWN, T. and VIRULRAK, S. (1991) 'Patterns of Bisexuality in Thailand', in TIELMAN, R., CARBALLO, M. and HENDRIKS, A. (Eds) *Bisexuality and HIV/AIDS: A Global Perspective*, New York, Prometheus.

TAN, M. L. (1994) 'From *Bakla* to Gay: Shifting Gender Identities and Sexual Behaviours in the Philippines', in PARKER, R. and GAGNON, J. (Eds) *Conceiving Sexuality: Approaches to Sex Research in a Postmodern World*, New York and London, Routledge.

TIGLAO, T. V. (1991) *Philippina KABP/PR Survey*, unpublished report, Manila.

# Notes on Contributors

**Peter Aggleton** is Professor in Education, Director of the Thomas Coram Research Unit and Associate Director of the Health and Education Research Unit at the Institute of Education, University of London. He has worked internationally in HIV/AIDS health promotion, and is currently coordinating a major programme of social and behavioural research for the World Health Organization's Global Programme on AIDS. His publications include *Deviance* (Tavistock, 1987); *Health* (Routledge, 1990); *AIDS: Rights, Risk and Reason* (Ed. with Peter Davies and Graham Hart, Taylor & Francis, 1992); *AIDS: Facing the Second Decade* (Ed. with Peter Davies and Graham Hart, Taylor & Francis, 1993); *AIDS: Foundations for the Future* (Ed. with Peter Davies and Graham Hart, Taylor & Francis, 1994); and *AIDS: Safety, Sexuality and Risk* (Ed. with Peter Davies and Graham Hart, Taylor & Francis, 1995).

**Dan Allman** is a sociologist and Research Coordinator within the HIV Social, Behavioural and Epidemiological Studies Unit of the University of Toronto, Canada. His current work focuses primarily on areas of human sexuality, specifically in regard to men who have sex with men. Additional fields of inquiry include health service and self-help organizations, communication technologies, multiculturalism and community-based research. He is author of numerous academic papers and presentations, and co-author (with Ted Myers and Rhonda Cockerill) of *Concepts, Definitions and Models for Community-Based HIV Prevention Research in Canada* (Ottawa, Health Canada, 1996).

**Mary Boulton** is Senior Lecturer in Sociology as Applied to Medicine at St Mary's Hospital Medical School (Imperial College), University of London. She has worked extensively investigating the factors contributing to the sexual behaviour of gay and bisexual men in relation to HIV/AIDS and is currently involved in research on the experience of families with an HIV-infected child and on the social aspects of genetic screening. She is editor of *Challenge and Innovation: Methodological Advances in Social Research on HIV/AIDS* (Taylor & Francis, 1994).

**Carlos F. Cáceres** is an assistant professor of public health and sexual/repro-ductive health at the Department of Public Health, and a research associate at the Institute of Population Studies at Cayetano Heredia University in Lima, Peru. He has broad research experience on sexuality and AIDS, where he combines epidemiological and sociocultural perspectives. He has worked with young people, men who have sex with other men and persons living with HIV/AIDS.

**June Crawford** is a Research Consultant to the National Centre in HIV Social Research at Macquarie University, Australia, where she has been involved in HIV/AIDS research since 1987. Her background is in social psychology and research methodology. She currently divides her research interests between the Sydney Men and Sexual Health (SMASH) cohort study and a project documenting the experiences of women living with HIV. Recent publications have appeared in *Feminism and Psychology* and *Venereology*.

**E. Antonio de Moya** is a psychologist and epidemiologist trained at Puerto Rican, North American, and Israeli universities. He headed the AIDS Research Department of the Dominican Republic's National AIDS Program from 1985 to 1993, and is presently a Research Associate at the Human Sexuality Institute of the Autonomous University of Santo Domingo in the Dominican Republic.

**Ray Fitzpatrick** is a Fellow of Nuffield College, Oxford, and University Lecturer in Medical Sociology at the University of Oxford. He has worked on a number of studies of gay and bisexual behaviour in relation to HIV/AIDS. Recent publications include *Measurement of Patients' Satisfaction with their Care* (Ed. with Anthony Hopkins, Royal College of Physicians, London, 1993); *Quality of Life in Health Care* (Ed. with Gary Albrecht, JAI Press, 1994) and *Understanding Rheumatoid Arthritis* (with Stan Newman, Tracey Revenson, Suzanne Skevington and Gareth Williams, Routledge, 1995).

**Rafael García** is a psychiatrist and sexologist trained at Dominican, British, and North American universities. He is a member of the Royal College of Psychiatrists of England, and Associate Fellow of the American Academy of Clinical Sexologists. Presently, he heads the Masters Programme of the Human Sexuality Institute at the Autonomous University of Santo Domingo in the Dominican Republic.

**Miguel Gonzáles Block** works at the National Institute of Public Health, Cuerrnavaca, and the Mexican Foundation for Health.

**Carol L. Jenkins** is Principal Research Fellow at the Papua New Guinea Institute of Medical Research and has conducted medical anthropological studies in Papua New Guinea for over a decade. She has worked on issues of sexual health and the risk of AIDS among sex workers, truckers, sailors, youth, and the rural population. She is currently conducting baseline research on HIV-related risk among youth in Fiji, West Samoa and elsewhere in the Pacific and coordinates an intervention among transport and sex workers in urban Papua New Guinea.

**Shivananda Khan** is the founder and Chief Executive of The Naz Project, an HIV/AIDS and Sexual Health agency for South Asian, Turkish, Arab and Irani communities, based in the UK. He is a founder member of The Naz Foundation (India) Trust based in New Delhi, India, developing sexual health programmes and HIV/AIDS support services. He has organized a range of training programmes, conferences and seminars in the UK, South Asia and elsewhere on HIV/AIDS and sexual behaviours.

**Susan Kippax** is Associate Professor in the School of Behavioural Sciences at Macquarie University, Australia. She has been involved in many aspects of HIV/AIDS research since 1986, and since 1990 has been the deputy director of the Australian National Centre in HIV Social Research. She is the author of numerous publications on the social aspects of AIDS, most recently in *AIDS*. She is also co-author of *Emotion and Gender: Constructing Meaning from Memory* (Sage, 1992).

**Ana Luisa Liguori** is an anthropologist and worked for over twenty years in the Department of Ethnology and Social Anthropology and History. Currently she is the country coordinator for the Fund for Leadership Development grants of the Population Program at the John D. and Catherine T. MacArthur Foundation in their Mexico office.

**Johnny Madrigal** is Executive Director of the Instituto Latinamericano de Educación y Prevención en Salud in San José, Costa Rica. He is a specialist researcher in the fields of sexuality and fertility, and is the co-author of *Primeir Encuesta Nacional Sobre Sida (en Costa Rica)* (Asociación Demográfica Costarricense, 1990) and *Hombres que aman Hombres* (Ilep-Sida, 1991).

**Antoine Messiah** works within the French National Institute for Health and Medical Research (INSERM) as a behavioural epidemiologist. He is a principal investigator with the French national survey on sexual behaviour.

**Ted Myers** is an Associate Professor in the Department of Health Administration and Director of the HIV Social, Behavioural and Epidemiological Studies Unit of the University of Toronto, Canada. His work has involved a variety of community-based AIDS/HIV evaluation and research programmes among gay and bisexual men, First Nations Peoples, injection drug users and prison populations. He has published numerous articles and presented papers at international conferences in the areas of addictions, HIV, health education, health promotion and health policy.

**Suiming Pan** is Professor and Head of the Institute for Research in Sexuality and Gender at Renmin University of China, Beijing. He has conducted research on sexuality and gender in China since 1982, including studies of HIV-related risk for the Ford Foundation and the Chinese National Sciences Foundation. He is the author of four books and numerous academic papers.

**Richard G. Parker** is Professor of Medical Anthropology and Human Sexuality in the Institute of Social Medicine at the State University of Rio de Janeiro, Brazil. Over the past decade, his work has focused on the social and cultural construction of gender and sexuality, as well as on the social aspects of HIV/AIDS. He is author of *Bodies, Pleasures and Passions: Sexual Culture in Contemporary Brazil* (Boston, Beacon Press, 1991) and co-author, with Herbert Daniel, of *Sexuality, Politics and AIDS in Brazil* (Taylor & Francis, 1993), and co-editor, with John H. Gagnon, of *Conceiving Sexuality: Approaches to Sex Research in a Postmodern World* (New York and London, Routledge, 1995).

**Garrett Prestage** is a Senior Research Fellow in the National Centre in HIV Social Research at Macquarie University, both in Sydney, Australia, and the National Centre in HIV Epidemiology and Clinical Research, University of New South Wales. He is the coordinator of the Sydney Men and Sexual Health cohort study which is a joint project of these two National Centres. He has a long involvement in Australian research on homosexually active men who do not identify as gay or homosexual.

**Jacobo Schifter** is Regional Director of the Instituto Latinamericano de Educación y Prevención en Salud in San José, Costa Rica and President of the Central American Confederation of NGOs against AIDS. He has published several books of Costa Rican and Central American history and is the author of *La Formación de una Contracultura: Homosexualismo y Sida en Costa Rica* (1989) and co-author of *Hombres que aman Hombres* (Ilep-Sida, 1992). He has written numerous articles on the social aspects of AIDS.

**Michael L. Tan** is a medical anthropologist. He is executive director of the Health Action Information Network and is Assistant Professor at the University of the Philippines. He is active with various organizations working in HIV/AIDS prevention and is a member of the Philippine National AIDS Council.

# Index